A ARUNPRASATH
GOPALAKRISHNAN THANGAVEL

Oral Mucosal Lesions in Dermatological Diseases

A ARUNPRASATH
GOPALAKRISHNAN THANGAVEL

Oral Mucosal Lesions in Dermatological Diseases

Cutaneous Diseases with Oral Involvement

LAP LAMBERT Academic Publishing

Imprint
Any brand names and product names mentioned in this book are subject to trademark, brand or patent protection and are trademarks or registered trademarks of their respective holders. The use of brand names, product names, common names, trade names, product descriptions etc. even without a particular marking in this work is in no way to be construed to mean that such names may be regarded as unrestricted in respect of trademark and brand protection legislation and could thus be used by anyone.

Cover image: www.ingimage.com

Publisher:
LAP LAMBERT Academic Publishing
is a trademark of
Dodo Books Indian Ocean Ltd. and OmniScriptum S.R.L publishing group

120 High Road, East Finchley, London, N2 9ED, United Kingdom
Str. Armeneasca 28/1, office 1, Chisinau MD-2012, Republic of Moldova, Europe
Managing Directors: Ieva Konstantinova, Victoria Ursu
info@omniscriptum.com

Printed at: see last page
ISBN: 978-620-9-51830-0

Dermatology, the specialized study of skin diseases, has become an important subdivision of the practice of medicine not only because of the many primary diseases that affect the skin, but also because of the common cutaneous manifestations of deeper visceral or systemic diseases. [1]

Dermatological diseases, besides involving the skin and its appendages may also involve the oral cavity. The lesions of oral cavity in dermatological disorders deserve special attention considering that they may be the presenting clinical feature or the only sign of these disorders. Moreover, oral mucosal lesions in skin diseases can be life-threatening and also affect the quality of life in terms of pain, discomfort, social and functional limitations. [2]

Significance for dentists: It is especially important for the dentist to recognize not only that some dermatological diseases but also exhibit concomitant lesions of the oral mucous membranes, but also that manifestation of some of the diseases may be preceded by oral lesions. Thus, the dentist may be in a position to establish the diagnosis of a dermatologic disease before the cutaneous lesions become apparent. [1]

Various groups of dermatological diseases associated with OML are, Infections, Vesiculobullous disorders, Lichen planus and other lichenoid disorders. Pemphigus vulgaris, lichen planus, candidiasis and recurrent apthous ulcers were the most frequently diagnosed conditions. [2]

The group of Vesiculobullous disorders includes viral diseases, autoimmune mucocutaneous diseases, diseases that probably have an immunologically mediated mechanism, and genetic diseases. The diagnosis of Vesiculobullous diseases should be made on clinical, histopathological, and immunological grounds. [3]

Mucosal disorders may be diagnosed from brief history and rapid clinical examination, but this approach is most often insufficient and leads to incorrect diagnosis and improper treatment. The history taking is frequently underemphasized, but, when correctly performed, it gives as much information as does the clinical examination. [3]

A complete review of systems should be obtained for each patient, including questions regarding the presence of skin, eye, genital, and rectal lesions. Questions should also be included regarding symptoms of diseases associated with oral lesions; that is, each patient should be asked about the presence of symptoms such as joint pains, muscle weakness, dyspnea, diplopia and chest pains. The clinical examination should include a thorough inspection of the exposed skin surfaces as the diagnosis of oral lesions requires knowledge of basic dermatologic lesions because many disorders occurring on the oral mucosa also affect the skin. [3]

Mucocutaneous disease (muco: Mucous membrane, cutaneous: Skin) are skin diseases that involves mucous membrane such as oral mucous membrane, genital mucosa etc. Skin has dual role (i.e) First, it forms a protective covering barrier and second, it also act as a part of the specialized immune apparatus of the body. Immune disturbances that forms a substantial part of disease pathogenesis are more commonly reflected in the skin as compared with other organ systems of the body. [3]

Oral cavity encompasses a diverse group of anatomical structures, including teeth and oral mucous membranes. An oral mucosal lesion (OML) is defined as any abnormal change or any swelling on the oral mucosal surface. It may be a result of local pathology or secondary to other systemic disease, including those of skin. In oral medicine, dermatological diseases have significance as OML may be primary clinical feature or the only sign of these disorders. A prevalence of 35% of OML in patients affected with dermatological conditions has been observed. [2]

This book will include the definitions, classifications, etiology, clinical features, histopathological features, diagnosis and treatment plan of all mucocutaneous disorders of the oral cavity.

CLASSIFICATIONS:

No Complete or Satisfactory classification is available for Mucocutaneous Disorders.

1) Vesicullobullous lesions it is classified according to their aetiology as follows: [4]

A.) INFECTIONS:

1. VIRAL:

1. HSV - Herpes Simplex Virus type1 and type2
2. VZV:
   i) Chicken pox
   ii) Zoster
3. Hand, Foot and mouth disease
4. Herpangina
5. Foot and Mouth Disease

1. BACTERIAL:

1. Impetigo
2. Anthrax
3. Gonnorrhoea
4. Cat-scratch disease
5. FUNGAL:

1. South American Blastomycosis

B. SKIN DISEASES:

1. Pemphigus
2. Bullous Pemphigoid
3. Beningn mucous memberane pemphigoid
4. Lupus Erythematosus
5. Dermatitis Herpetiformis
6. Lichen Planus
7. Erythema Multiforme and Stephens - Johnson Syndrome
8. Toxic Epidermal Necrolysis
9. Epidermolysis Bullosa
10. Dyskeratosis Congenita

C. DRUG-INDUCED:

1. Empepronium Bromide
2. Sulphonamides
3. Phenolphthalein
4. Phenacitin
5. Chloroquine
6. Arsenic
7. Mercury
8. Phenylbutazone

D. MISCELLANEOUS:

1. Oral Sub Mucous Fibrosis - intial stages

2) CLASSIFICATION [2]

Various groups of dermatological diseases associated with OML are as follows:

• Infections

1. Herpes simplex
2. Varicella zoster virus
3. Herpangina
4. Hand, foot and mouth disease
5. Oral hairy leukoplakia
6. HIV Infection
7. Oral candidosis
8. Syphilis
9. Leprosy
10. Leishmaniasis

• Vesicobullous disorders

11. Pemphigus vulgaris
12. Paraneoplastic pemphigus
13. Mucous membrane pemphigoid
14. Epidermolysis bullosa

Connective tissue disorders

15. Systemic lupus erythemotosus.
16. Systemic sclerosis
17. Sjögren's syndrome

• Lichen planus and other lichenoid disorders:

18. Lichen planus
19. Contact Stomatitis/ Contact Lichenoid reaction

Collagen vascular diseases

• Vasculitis

20. Kawasaki disease
21. Behçet's disease
22. Wegener's granulomatosis

• Genodermatosis

23. Tuberous sclerosis complex
24. Ectodermal dysplasias

• Miscellaneous

- Erythema multiforme
- Stevens–johnson syndrome
- Toxic epidermal necrolysis
- Angio-oedema
- Sarcoidosis
- Langerhans'cell histiocytosis (LCH)

3) CLASSIFICATION OF ORAL LESIONS [5]

Reactive oral lesions were histologically classified using Neville's classification of common mucosal overgrowth.

Lesions were classified as:

Hyperplastic lesions

1. Fibroepithelial hyperplasia
2. Irritation fibroma
3. Epulis fissuratum
4. Fibrous polyps
5. Cheek-biting lesions

Reactive

6. Peripheral giant cell granuloma
7. Pyogenic granuloma
8. Peripheral ossifying fibroma
9. Giant cell fibroma

Non neoplastic pigmented lesions

10. Amalgam tattoo
11. Melanosis
12. Melanotic macule.

Dermatoses:

13. Pemphigus vulgaris
14. Mucous membrane pemphigoid
15. Lupus erythematosus
16. Bullous pemphigoid

Lichen planus:

17. Bullous lichen planus
18. Erosive lichen planus
19. Lichenoid reactions

Nonspecific inflammatory lesions:

20. Epulis granulomatosa
21. Benign and malignant tumors are also included.
22.

4) CLASSIFICATION OF SKIN DISEASES:

ANDRWS AND REGEZI CLASSIFICATION: [6]

1) Congenital ectodermal defects:

1. Hypohidrotic ectodermal dysplasia (anhidrotic ectodermal dysplasia)
2. Hidrotic ectodermal dysplasia (clouston syndrome)

2) Immune mediated diseases:

a) Lichen planus:

1. Linear lichen planus
2. Annular lichen planus
3. Hypertrophic lichen planus
4. Ulcerative lichen planus

5. Bullous lichen planus
6. Follicular lichen planus
7. Drug induced lichen planus

b) Reiter's syndrome

c) Graft versus host disease

d) Systemic sclerosis

e) CREST syndrome

f) Papulosquamous dermatoses

g) Psoriasis

h) Pityriasis rosea

3) Chronic blistering dermatoses:

a) Pemphigus

1. Pemphigus vulgaris
2. Pemphiogus vegetans
3. Pemphigus foliaceus
4. Brazilian pemphigus
5. Pemphigus erythematosus

b) Paraneoplastic pemphigus

c) Cicartricial pemphigoid

d) Epidermolysis bullosa acquisita

e) Dermatitis herpetiformis

4) Vesicles/bullae/pustules

a) Erythema and urticaria

1. Erythema multiforme
2. Erythema migrans
3. Drug induced bullous erythema multiforme
4. Toxic epidermal necrolysis
5. Annular urticarial reactions

5) Endocrine diseeases:

- Acanthosis nigrans

6) Connective tissue diseases

- Lupus erythematosus

7) Some genodermatosis and acquired syndromes:

1. Epidermolysis bullosa
2. Pachyonychia congenital
3. Darier;s disease
4. Hailey hailey disease
5. Incontinentia pigmenti
6. Dyskeratosis congenital
7. Porokeratosis

8) Epidermal nevi

- White sponge nevus

9) Dermatoses resulting from physical factors

- Solar elastosis

10) Abnormalities of dermal connective tissue

-Ehlers danlos syndrome

5) CLASSIFICATION: [7]

Classification of VesicculloBullous Diseases:

A. Acute and Chronic Vesicullo Bullous Lesions:

Acute:

1. Chicken pox,
2. Herpes Simplex,
3. Herpes Zoster,
4. Herpangina,
5. Hand Foot and Mouth disease,
6. Erythema Multiforme

Chronic:

1. Pemphigus,
2. Bullous Pemphigoid,
3. Cicatrial Pemphigoid,
4. Bullous Lichen planus,
5. Chronic Herpes Simplex,
6. Linear IgA disease,

B. Based on Clinical Presentation:

1. Predominantly Vesicular:

1. HSV infection
2. Varicella infection
3. Hand Foot and Mouth diasease
4. Herpangina
5. Dermatitis Herpetiformis

2. Predominantly Bullous:
1. Pemphigus Vulgaris
2. Bullous Pemphigoid
3. Benign Mucous Memberane Pemphigoid,
4. Bullous Lichen Planus,
5. Erythema Multiforme,
6. Stephens-Johnson syndrome,
7. Bullous Impetigo,

Epidermolysis Bullosa,

1. Linear IgA Disease.

C. Histopathological Classification:

1. Intra Epithelial Vesicullo Bullous Lesions:
1. HSV Infection
2. Varicella Infection
3. Herpangina
4. Hand Foot Mouth Disease
5. Pemphigus
6. Familial Benign Chronic Pemphigus
7. Epidermolysis Bullosa
8. Mucosal Erythema Multiforme

2. Sub Epithelial Vesicullobullous Lesions:
1. Bullous Pemphigoid
2. Cicatricial Pemphigoid
3. Epidermolysis Bullosa
4. Dermal Erythema Multiforme
5. Dermatitis Herpetiformis
6. Linear IgA Disease

D. Based on whether the lesions are infectious or Non Infectious:

Infectious Vesicullo Bullous Lesions:

1. Herpes Simplex Infections
2. Varicella Infections
3. Herpangina
4. Hand Foot And Mouth Disease

Non Infectious Vesicullo Bullous Lesions:

1. Pemphigus
2. Para Neoplastic Pemphigus
3. Bullous Pemphigoid
4. Cicatricial Pemphigoid
5. Erythema Multiforme
6. Dermatitis Herpetiformans
7. Epidermolysis Bullosa Acquisita
8. Linear IgA Disease

6. CLASSIFICATION: [2]

Based on Infections:

1. Herpes simplex
2. Herpangina
3. Varicella zoster virus
4. Hand, foot and mouth disease
5. Oral hairy leukoplakia
6. HIV Infection
7. Oral candidiasis
8. Syphilis
9. Leprosy
10. Leishmaniasis

Based on Vesiculo-bullous disorders:

1. Pemphigus vulgaris
2. Paraneoplastic pemphigus
3. Mucous membrane pemphigoid
4. Epidermolysis bullosa

Based on Connective tissue disorders:

1. Systemic lupus erythematosus
2. Systemic sclerosis
3. Sjogren's syndrome

Based on Lichenoid dermatosis:

1. Lichen planus
2. Contact Stomatitis/ Contact Lichenoid reaction

Based on Vasculitis:

1. Kawasaki disease
2. Behçet's disease
3. Wegener's granulomatosis

Based on Genodermatosis:

1. Tuberous sclerosis complex
2. Ectodermal dysplasias

Miscellaneous:

1. Erythema multiforme,
2. Stevens–johnson syndrome and
3. Toxic epidermal necrolysis

TERMINOLOGIES: [8]

1. Macules:

These are well-circumscribed, flat lesions that are noticeable because of their change from normal skin or mucosa color. They may be red due to increased vascularity or inflammation, or pigmented due to the presence of melanin, hemosiderin, and foreign material or ingestion of medications. A good example in the oral cavity is the melanotic macule.

2. Papules:

These are solid lesions raised above the skin or mucosal surface that are smaller than 1 cm in diameter. Papules may be seen in a wide variety of diseases, including erythema multiforme, rubella, lupus erythematosus, and sarcoidosis. In the oral cavity hyperplastic candidiasis often presents as yellow-white papules.

3. Plaques:

These are solid raised lesions that are greater than 1cm in diameter; they are large papules.

4. Nodules:

These lesions are present deeper in the dermis or mucosa. The lesions may also protrude above the skin or mucosa but are generally wider than they are high. A good example of an oral mucosal nodule is the irritation fibroma.

5. Vesicles:

These are elevated blisters containing clear fluid that are less than 1 cm in diameter.

6. Bullae:

These are elevated blisters containing clear fluid that are greater than 1cm in diameter.

7. Erosions:

These are red lesions often caused by the rupture of vesicles or bullae or trauma and are generally moist on the skin.

8. Pustules:

These are blisters containing purulent material.

9. Ulcers:

These are well-circumscribed, often depressed lesions with an epithelial defect that is covered by a fibrin clot, causing a yellow-white appearance. A good example is an aphthous ulcer.

10. Purpura:

These are reddish to purple bruises caused by blood from vessels leaking into the connective tissue. These lesions do not blanch when pressure is applied and are classified by size as petechiae (less than 0.5 cm) or ecchymoses.

SECONDARY SKIN LESIONS: [6]

1. Scale:

Flaky exfoliation, a plate-like excrescence of varied size, usually composed of accumulated stratum corneum.

E.g.

- Psoriasis
- Dermatitis
- Tinea versicolor
- Pityriasis rosea.

2. Crust (scab):

A solid consolidation of dried serum, blood, pus.

E.g.

- Eczema
- Scab on abrasion.

3. Lichenification:

Thickened and rough epidermis with accentuation of skin markings.

E.g.

1. Chronic contact eczema.

4. Scar:

Fibrous tissue secondary to dermis injury. It may be pink, red or white; atrophic or hypertrophic (keloid).

E.g.

1. Healed wound.

5. Excoriation:

Loss of epidermis caused by a traumatic lesion causing a linear area.

E.g.

- Deep scratch
- Abrasion.

6. Fissure:

A linear and small split or crack in the epidermis and dermis.

E.g.

1. Cheilosis.

7. Erosion:

Discontinuity of the skin with loss of part or all epidermis, usually follows rupture of vesicle or bulla.

E.g.

- Varicella (following rupture)
- Variola (following rupture)

8. Ulceration:

Discontinuity of the skin with loss of epidermis; and sometimes hipodermis. Usually heals with scaring.

E.g.

- Decubitus
- Herpes ssimplex
- Syphilis (chancre).

9. Ulcers:

Ulceration without tendency of healing (scaring).

E.g.

1. Stasis ulcers.

10. Atrophy:

Reduction of skin thickening ocurring at any skin layer.

E.g.

- Striae
- Aged skin.

VASCULAR LESIONS: [6]

1. Purpura:

Red-purple nonblanching colored lesion due to extravation of blood into the tissue.

E.g.

- Henoch-Schönlein purpura
- Thrombocytopenic purpura

2. Petechiae:

It is a punctiform purpura.

E.g. • Vasculitis

- Infection.

3. Ecchymoses:

Purpura greater than 1 cm in diameter.

E.g.

- Trauma
- Vasculitis.

4. Telangiectasia:

Permanent dilated superficial blood vessels.

E.g.

- Telangiectasia in liver disease
- Telangiectasia in pregnancy
- Telangiectasia in breast cancer
- Telangiectasia in lupus erythematosus, systemic or discoid.

Mucocutaneous diseases are confined to the stratified squamous epithelium and thus may involve skin, oral and other mucosa like the nasal, ocular, genital mucosa.

An understanding of the basic molecular aspects of these disorders is essential for proper diagnosis. Once a definitive diagnosis is determined, treatment is focused upon the alleviation of clinical signs and symptoms, referral for consultation with other specialists to assess the extent of the disease process, and the prevention of recurrence. [9]

A. INFECTIONS:

1) VIRAL:

i) HERPES SIMPLEX VIRUS (HSV):

Etiopathogenesis:

The herpes viruses, including herpes simplex virus type one and type two, have the potential to initiate oral mucocutaneous lesions which are often painful and recurrent in nature. Most oral herpetic lesions are the result of herpes simplex type I infection. Most patients are exposed to the herpes simplex type I virus during the first five years of life, which usually results in nothing more than a subclinical infection. However, in approximately 5% of the population, this initial exposure results in primary herpetic gingivostomatitis. Following initial exposure, the virus follows neuronal pathways to immune privileged sites such as the trigeminal ganglion and a period of latency occurs. Although the mechanism remains unclear, reactivation of the virus may lead to the development of conditions such as recurrent herpetic stomatitis and herpes labialis. When recurrent lesions affect the oral cavity, they appear as multiple small vesicles that rupture, to form ulcerations which may coalesce to form larger lesions. In contrast to recurrent aphthous stomatitis, these lesions frequently occur on mucosa that is non-mobile such as the hard palate and attached gingiva. Occasionally precipitated by dental treatment, recurrent herpetic stomatitis lesions generally heal within 7 to 10 days. [10].

ii) VARICELLA ZOSTER VIRUS (VZV):

Etiopathogenesis:

Primary varicella-zoster virus (VZV) infections in sero negative individuals are known as varicella or chickenpox; secondary or reactivated disease is known as herpes zoster or shingles. Structurally, VZV is very similar to HSV, with a DNA core, a protein capsid, and a lipid envelope. Microscopically, striking similarities can also be noted. The ability of the virus to remain quiescent in sensory ganglia for indefinite periods after a primary infection is common to both. A cutaneous oro mucosal vesiculo-ulcerative eruption following reactivation of latent virus is also typical of both VZV and HSV infections. A number of signs and symptoms, however, appear to be unique to each infection. Transmission of varicella is believed to be predominantly through the inhalation of contaminated droplets. The condition is very contagious and is known to spread readily from child to child. Much less commonly, direct contact is an alternative way of acquiring the disease. During the 2-week incubation period, virus proliferates within macrophages, with subsequent viraemia and dissemination to the skin and other organs. Host defense mechanisms of nonspecific interferon production and specific humoral and cell-mediated immune responses are also triggered. Overt clinical disease then appears in most individuals. As the viremia overwhelms body defenses, systemic signs and symptoms develop. Eventually, in a normal host the immune response is able to limit and halt the replication of virus, allowing recovery in 2 to 3 weeks. During the disease process the VZV may progress along sensory nerves to the sensory ganglia, where it can reside in a latent, undetectable form. Reactivation of latent VZV is uncommon but characteristically follows such occurrences as immunosuppressive states resulting from malignancy (especially lymphomas and leukemias), drug administration, or HIV infection. Radiation or surgery of the spinal cord or local trauma may also trigger secondary lesions. [11]

iii) HAND-FOOT-AND-MOUTH DISEASE:

Etiopathogenesis:

Hand-foot-and-mouth disease is caused by a coxsackievirus, an Enterovirus. In most instances coxsackievirus type A16 has been isolated; only rarely has another type, such as A5 or A9, been found. Hand-foot-and-mouth disease occurs in small epidemics, affecting mainly children and having a mild course that usually lasts less than a week. Transmission is mainly via fecal -oral contact and less commonly by respiratory droplets. Symptoms usually appear 3 to 5 days after exposure. After a 1-to 2-day mild prodrome of low-grade fever, sore throat, and malaise, small red macules present on the oral mucosal and progress to 1- to 3-mm vesicles, where they evolve into small ulcers. [11]

iv) HERPANGINA:

Etiopathogenesis:

Herpangina is an acute viral infection caused by another Coxsackie type A virus (types A1-6, A8, A10, A22, B3, and possibly others). It is transmitted by contaminated saliva and occasionally through contaminated faeces. Herpangina is usually endemic, with outbreaks occurring typically in summer or early autumn. It is more common in children than in adults. Those infected generally complain of malaise, fever, dysphagia, and sore throat after a short incubation period. [11]

2) BACTERIAL:

i) IMPETIGO:

Etiopathogenesis:

Impetigo is a bacterial infection that affects the superficial areas of the skin. It commonly affects infants and young children in the age group of 2–5 years. However it has known to affect individuals of various age groups. It is a highly contagious infection caused primarily by Staphylococcus aureus. However some cases have been reportedly caused by group A beta-hemolytic streptococcus (Streptococcus pyogenes) alone or in tandem with Staphylococcus aureus. The mode of transmission is generally by direct contact. Bullous impetigo is usually seen in infants. But it is seen to affect children and adults likewise. Unlike the non bullous form which may be caused by a combination of staphylococcus and streptococcus. Bullous forms is always caused by the toxins produced by Staphylococcus aureus. Staphylococcus aureus, phage group II type 71 is the predominant causative organism. This strain of bacteria produces an exfoliatin toxin that causes sub corneal epidermal cleavage. The exotoxin produced by staphylococci is directed against epidermal desmoglein 1. [7]

ii) GONORRHOEA:

Etiopathogenesis:

The incidence of gonorrhea has increased in developing countries, but the exact incidence is difficult to ascertain because of limited surveillance and variable diagnostic criteria. It is transmitted from males to females and vice versa. Oropharyngeal gonorrhea occurs in 20% of women who practice fellatio with infected partners. The incubation period is one to five days. [1]

iii) CAT SCRATCH DISEASE:

Etiopathogenesis:

Though common in the USA and Britain, it is relatively rare in the Indian subcontinent. The causative organism is Bartonella henselae, a gram-negative bacillus demonstrable with silver stain. [1]

B. henselae infection accompanied by bacteremia, which can persist for more than a year. It is believed that domestic cats tend to rapidly develop antibodies and therefore appear healthy in spite of the bacteremia. The first description in the literature of cat-scratch disease is credited to Henri Parinaud in 1889. Dr Robert Debré in 1931 described a case of a boy with a cat-scratch on his hand associated with a suppurative epitrochlear lymph node. He is credited with recognizing the cat as the vector of this illness and coined the term 'catscratch disease'. Regnery and coworkers (1992) identified B. henselae as the causative organism for cat-scratch disease. Cat-scratch disease is considered as a self-limiting granulomatous condition characterized by suppurative regional lymphadenitis. [7]

3) FUNGAL:

Etiopathogenesis:

Blastomycosis was first described in America by the American dermatologist, Thomas Caspar Gilchrist in 1894. It is caused by Blastomyces dermatitidis, a dimorphic fungus. It is believed to thrive in organic matter and soil which have high moisture content. Following inhalation of the spores, three forms of the disease are manifested: acute, chronic and a disseminated form. [7]

4) CHLAMYDEAL:

Etiopathogenesis:

Lymphogranuloma venereum, a venereal disease that is caused by strains of chlamydia trachomatis. [1]

Chlamydia are minute gram negative cocci that are intracellular parasites. C. pneumonia has been recently implicated in atherosclerotic processes. There is a very high likelihood of human to human transmission of lymphogranuloma venereum through unprotected sexual activity. The primary lesion of lymphogranuloma venereum occurs in the anogenital region about 10 days after exposure and presents as a small vesicle, which ruptures and heals without scarring. About 1 week to 2 months later, swelling and tenderness of the regional lymph nodes occur, and suppuration via multiple sinuses may supervene. The large intestine may also become involved, and healing usually occurs with scar formation. [8]

B. SKIN DISEASES:

1) PEMPHIGUS VULGARIS:

Etiopathogenesis:

Pemphigus vulgaris is an autoimmune disorder in which there is deposition of mainly IgG class antibodies intracellularly, as well as damage to desmosomes by antibodies directed against the extracellular domains of cadherin-type epithelial cell adhesion molecules, particularly desmoglein 3 (DSG 3). Since oral epithelium largely expresses DSG 3 ; but skin expresses DSG 1 as well as DSG 3,damage to DSG 3 by antibodies results in oral lesions at an early stages but skin integrity maintained by DSG

.However, if damage to DSG 1 antibodies appear, cutanous lesions appear and the disease tends to be more severe. The appearance of serum antibodies against DSG 1 heralds involvement of skin and mucosa other than oral. The immune reaction against these glycoproteins causes a loss of cell to cell adhesion (ACANTHOLYSIS) resulting in the formation of INTRAEPITHELIAL BULLAE. The mechanism by which anti desmoglein antibodies cause the loss of cell-cell adhesion is controversial. Some believe the binding of the Pemphigus Vulgaris antibody activates proteases, whereas recently, it is considered that Pemphigus Vulgaris antibodies directly block the adhesion function of the desmogleins. [12]

1. BULLOUS PEMPHIGOID:

Etiopathogenesis:

Bullous Pemphigoid is a sub epidermal skin blistering disease characterized immunohistologically by dermal-epidermal junction separation, an infammatory cell infiltrate in the upper dermis, and autoantibodies targeted toward the hemidesmosomal proteins Bullous Pemphigoid 230 and Bullous Pemphigoid 180. Oral lesions begin as bullae, but they tend to rupture sooner, probably as a result of constant low-grade trauma to which the oral mucosa is subjected. Large, shallow ulcerations with smooth, distinct margins are present after the bullae rupture. Sometimes erosions are confined to the gingiva creating a picture of chronic desquamative gingivitis. [13]

3) MUCOUS MEMBRANE PEMPHIGOID:

Etiopathogenesis:

MMP is an autoimmune disorder, usually of unknown cause but occasionally triggered by drugs and occasionally associated with other autoimmune diseases. There may be no known racial or geographic predilections, but there may be an immunogenetic background and an association with HLA DQB1*0301 (Human Leucocyte

Antigen) which is especially notable in ocular pemphigoid. The pathophysiologic mechanism of MMP is complex and poorly understood. There is clearly a defect in the immune regulation involving the formation of autoantibodies directed against antigens, which are normal components of the basal membrane zone. The separation of the epithelium from the underlying tissue within the Basal membrane zone may be the result of a direct cytotoxic action or the effect of lysosomal proteolytic enzymes. Cellular immunity and cytokines also play a role in the pathogenesis of MMP. The cytokine tumor necrosis factor-alpha (TNF-α) is thought to play a prominent role in the pathogenesis of MMP. The chronic overproduction of TNF-α was recently implicated in the pathogenesis of MMP and other autoimmune blistering disorders. Consequently, MMP may not be a distinct disease entity but, rather, a series of syndromes with different causes and pathogenetic mechanisms. [12]

The pathogenesis of MMP can best be understood by considering the normal epithelial–connective tissue interface. Autoantibodies (IgG or IgA or both) attack 1 or more antigen sites in the molecules connecting the epithelium to the connective tissue and prevent the linkage of molecules in the hemidesmosomes. The major antigens involved in oral MMP are believed to be and laminin 512,13 (Fig. 2f). Consequently, the epithelium is poorly anchored to the connective tissue and separates, allowing a subepithelial blister to form. There is evidence to show that the severity of the disease is proportional to the concentration of autoantibodies and the number of classes of antibodies involved (i.e., both IgG and IgA). [14]

4) LUPUS ERYTHEMATOSUS:

Etiopathogenesis:

Bullous systemic lupus erythematosus (BSLE) is a rare variant of systemic lupus erythematosus (SLE) which histologically resembles dermatitis herpetiformis (DH) and responds dramatically to dapsone. BSLE is an autoantibody mediated subepidermal blistering disease that occurs in patients with SLE. Not all blistering eruptions that occur in patients with lupus erythematosus represent BSLE. Vesiculo-bullous skin lesions can also develop as a result of extensive damage to the epidermal basal layer (and even suprabasal keratinocytes) due to intense interface dermatitis in the setting of lupus erythematosus specific skin disease. Such patients may present with a severe form of acute or subacute cutaneous lupus erythematosus (SCLE) that resembles erythema multiforme (Rowell syndrome) or TEN. Because SCLE and BSLE share the same target antigen, distinguishing between the two may be difficult. [11]

5) DERMATITIS HERPETIFORMIS:

Etiopathogenesis:

Dermatitis herpetiformis is a cutaneous vesiculo-bullous disease characterized by intense pruritus. The disease is associated with granular IgA deposits in the papillary dermis that precipitate with an epidermal trans-glutaminase, an enzyme not normally present in the papillary region of normal skin. Serum IgA in patients with dermatitis herpetiformis also binds epidermal transglutaminase. Dermatitis herpetiformis is frequently associated with the gluten-sensitive enteropathy, celiac disease, which is characterized by IgA type autoantibodies to a closely related enzyme, tissue transglutaminase. It is now widely accepted that dermatitis herpetiformis is a cutaneous manifestation of celiac disease and affects approximately 25% of patients with celiac disease. Both dermatitis herpetiformis and celiac disease are closely linked to Human leucocyte antigen (HLA class II locus in chromosome 6 with 90% of patients having HLA DQ2 and almost all the remainder HLA DQ8). [11]

6. ORAL LICHEN PLANUS:

Etiopathogenesis:

The exact etiology is not known. However, OLP is a T-cell mediated auto-immune disorder in which auto-cytotoxic CD8 T cells triggers the apoptosis of oral epithelial cells, leading to chronic inflammation. [12]

7) ERYTHEMA MULTIFORME:

Etiopathogenesis:

Although the etiology of erythema multiforme is not fully understood, many cases are believed to be related to allergic or hypersensitivity reactions. A variety of medications, including sulfonamides, have been implicated as potential causative factors. In addition, many episodes of erythema multiforme are preceded by bacterial or viral infections such as mycoplasma pneumonia and herpes simplex lesions, suggesting a hypersensitivity reaction to an antigenic component of one of these microorganisms. As a result, a careful history of recent illnesses and medications can provide clues to aid in the prevention of recurrence experienced by 25% of affected patients. [10]

Erythema multiforme appears to be the result of a cell-mediated immune reaction to the precipitating agent. In EM, it is most likely that HSV– DNA fragments in the skin or mucosa precipitate the disease. HSV–DNA fragments and in particular DNA polymerase (PoL) have been detected in the basal and suprabasal cell layers of the epidermis in lesions as well as healed lesions for upto 3 months and the T cell accumulating in active lesions are CD4+ (Vb2+) cells which respond to HSV antigens in vitro. In addition, there is a good correlation between PoL expression in lesions, CD4+ (Vb2+) T cell accumulation and the duration of clinical symptoms. In situ Polymerase Chain Reaction and immunocytochemical staining have shown that mononuclear cells in both EM and HSV lesional skin tissues stain positively for Interferon-c (IFN), a cytokine, which is associated with tissue damage, and this expression correlates with HSV-protein expression. IFN-c is produced by CD4+ T helper 1 (Th1) lymphocytes, cells characteristic of a delayed type hypersensitivity reaction. IFN-c is proinflammatory and induces adhesion molecule expression on keratinocytes and endothelial cells as well as stimulating production of chemokines and cytokines from a number of cell types. Thus, it seems likely that the HSV–DNA fragments in skin or mucosa initiate a specific T-cell mediated response resulting in the presence of HSV-specific T cells, which generate IFN-c. This cytokine then amplifies the immune response and stimulates the production of additional cytokines and chemokines, which aids the recruitment of further reactive T cells to the area. These cytotoxic T cells, NK cells or chemokines can all induce epithelial damage. The mechanisms of tissue damage in EM appear to differ between virally induced and drug-induced EM and also differ from those in SJS and TEN, particularly those that are characterized by widespread epithelial damage but with a sparse inflammatory infiltrate. [6]

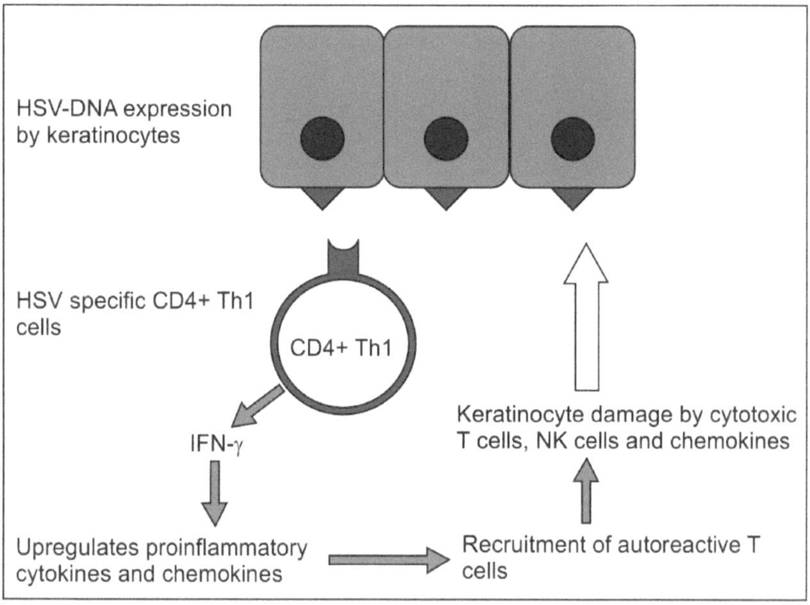

8) TOXIC EPIDERMAL NECROLYSIS (TEN):

Etiopathogenesis:

Toxic epidermal necrolysis (TEN) and Stevens Johnson Syndrome (SJS) are severe adverse cutaneous drug reactions that predominantly involve the skin and mucous membranes. Drugs are assumed or identified as the main cause of SJS/TEN in most cases, but Mycoplasma pneumoniae and Herpes simplex virus infections are well documented causes alongside rare cases in which the aetiology remains unknown. Several drugs are at "high" risk of inducing TEN/SJS including: Allopurinol, Trimethoprim-sulfamethoxazole and other sulfonamide-antibiotics, aminopenicillins, cephalosporins, quinolones, carbamazepine, phenytoin, phenobarbital and NSAID's of the oxicam-type. Genetic susceptibility to SJS and TEN is likely as exemplified by the strong association observed in Han Chinese between a genetic marker, the human leukocyte antigen HLA-B*1502, and SJS induced by carbamazepine. [11]

9) EPIDERMOLYSIS BULLOSA:

Etiopathogenesis:

Epidermolysis bullosa is a general term that encompasses one acquired and several genetic varieties (dystrophic, junctional, and simplex) of disease that are basically characterized by the formation of blisters at sites of minor trauma. The several genetic types range from autosomal dominant to autosomal recessive in origin and are further distinguished by various clinical features, histopathology, and ultrastructure. The acquired nonhereditary autoimmune form, known as epidermolysis acquisita, is unrelated to the other types and is often precipitated by exposure to specific drugs. In this type, IgG deposits are commonly found in sub-basement membrane tissue and type VII collagen antibodies located below the lamina densa of the basement membrane. In the hereditary forms of epidermolysis bullosa, circulating antibodies are not evident. Rather, pathogenesis appears to be related to genetic defects in basal cells, hemidesmosomes, or anchoring connective tissue filaments, depending on the disease subtype. [11]

10) DYSKERATOSIS CONGENITA:

Etiopathogenesis:

Mutations in DKC 1(Dyskeratosis Congenita) have been shown to cause the X-linked form of DKC. The inheritance pattern of most cases of DKC is X-linked recessive, but autosomal dominant and recessive patterns have been reported. [3]

It is a pre-malignant condition. It is genetically heterogeneous, with X-linked recessive, autosomal dominant and autosomal recessive subtypes. It is related to telomerase dysfunction. Telomeres are repeat structures found at the ends of chromosomes that function to stabilize chromosomes. With each round of cell division, the length of telomeres is shortened and the enzyme telomerase compensates by maintaining telomere length in germline and stem cells. Because telomeres function to maintain chromosomal stability, telomerase has a critical role in preventing cellular senescence and cancer progression. Rapidly proliferating tissues with the greatest need for telomere maintenance (e.g. bone marrow) are at greatest risk for failure. [7]

C) DRUG INDUCED:

1) LICHENOID REACTION:

Etiopathogenesis:

The exact mechanism of the development of lichenoid reaction (LR) is not known, but a series of triggering factors, such as dental restorative materials, graft-versus-host disease, a broad range of drugs, flavoring agents, and tobacco chewing are identified in the causation of LR. Drugs such as antimalarials, non-steroidal anti-inflammatory drugs, antihypertensive agents, oral hypoglycemics, and beta blockers were reported to be associated with LR. Scully and Diz Dios have reported oral lichenoid reactions associated with antiretroviral therapy in HIV infection. Dental restorative materials such as silver amalgam, gold, cobalt, palladium, chromium and epoxy resins, preservatives and flavoring agents commonly used in foods and dentifrices also trigger LR. Contact hypersensitivity to dental restorative materials was attributed to galvanism in the past. But recent studies have suggested a cell mediated contact hypersensitivity to dental materials in the susceptible individuals, and the contact allergy to dental materials mostly involves type IV delayed hypersensitivity reaction. Oral lichenoid reactions are considered to be a part of the spectrum of graft-versus host disease. Daftary and coworkers as early as in 1980 reported lichen planus-like lesion in tobacco chewers. [1]

TABLE 1: [15]

Anticholinergics

(i) Solifenacin

Anticonvulsants

(i) Carbamazepine

(ii) Oxcarbazepine

(iii) Phenytoin

(iv)Valproate sodium

Antidiabetics

(i) Chlorpropamide

(ii) Glyburide

(iii) Glipizide

(iv) Insulin

(v) Tolazamide

(vi) Tolbutamide

Antidiarrheals

(i) Bismuth

Antigout

(i) Allopurinol

Antihistamine drugs

(i) Cinnarizine

(ii) Iodides

Anti-inflammatory drugs

(i) Aspirin

(ii) Diflunisal

(iii) Ibuprofen

(iv) Indomethacin

(v) Leflunomide

(vi) Mesalamine

(vii) Naproxen

(viii) Rofecoxib

(ix) Sulindac

(x) Sulfasalazine

(xi) Tolbutamide

Antimalarials

(i) Chloroquine

(ii) Hydroxychloroquine

(iii) Pyrimethamine

(iv) Quinidine

(v) Quinine

Antimicrobials

Antibiotics

(i) Para-aminosalicylic acid

(ii) Sulphamethoxazole

(iii) Tetracycline

Antimycobacterials

(i) Aminosalicylate sodium

(ii) Dapsone

(iii) Ethambutol

(iv) Isoniazid

(v) Rifampin

(vi) Streptomycin

Antifungals

(i) Amphotericin B

(ii) Griseofulvin

(iii) Ketoconazole

Antihelminthic

(i) Levamisole

Antiparkinsonian drugs

(i) Trihexyphenidyl

Antiretrovirals

(i) Zidovudine

Chemotherapy drugs

(i) Hydroxyurea

Other medications

(i) Amiphenazole

(ii) Clopidogrel

(iii) Penacillamine

(iv) Palifermin

(v) Mercapto-propionylglycine

(vi) Misoprostol

(vii) Nandrolene

(viii) Furyl-propionate (Demelon)

(ix) Norflex

(x) Omeprazole

(xi) Pyrithioxin

(xii) Sildenafil

(xiii) Tiopronin

2) PEMPHIGUS FOLIACEUS:

Etiopathogenesis:

Pemphigus foliaceus (PF) is generally a benign variety of pemphigus. It is an autoimmune skin disorder characterized by the loss of intercellular adhesion of keratinocytes in the upper parts of the epidermis (acantholysis), resulting in the formation of superficial blisters. It includes the following six subtypes: pemphigus erythematosus (PE), pemphigus herpetiformis (PH), endemic pemphigus foliaceus, immunoglobulin A (IgA) pemphigus foliaceus, paraneoplastic pemphigus foliaceus (PNPF), and drug-induced pemphigus foliaceus. [1]

3) DRUG INDUCED ERYTHEMA MULTIFORME:

Etiopathogenesis:

In drug induced EM, it is thought that reactive metabolites of the initiating drug induce the disease but the mechanisms of damage are variable and unlike EM do not appear to be the result of a immune response. Immuno cytochemicial staining and in situ hybridization has shown that T cells do not produce IFN-g in drug-induced lesions but rather the lesions are characterized by tumor necrosis factor alpha (TNF-α) present in keratinocytes and also produced by macrophages and monocytes. In contrast, TNF-α has not been detected in EM and it has even been proposed that its presence may be used as a laboratory test to distinguish drug-induced lesions from EM . Much of the tissue damage in drug-induced lesions appears to be due to apoptosis and, because of the paucity of the inflammatory reaction; attention has recently been focused on soluble factors and cytokines. Locally produced TNF-α may be important since, it has been shown to mediate keratinocyte apoptosis and it is possible this mechanism plays a role in milder forms of drug-induced EM. However, particularly in TEN and SJS, there is some evidence for a gene Fas–FasL interaction. FasL mediates apoptotic cell death by binding to Fas on cells and inducing the formation of caspases. Fas is present on keratinocytes and FasL is found on activated T cells and NK cells and thus binding of keratinocytes to T cells or NK (Natural Killer) cells can induce apoptosis. One report suggests that keratinocytes in TEN may express FasL, which could potentially induce cell death in a neighbouring keratinocyte but it is not clear whether such a mechanism is generally operative. There is also evidence that soluble FasL (sFasL) produced by peripheral blood mononuclear cells may be important, since high levels of sFasL are present in the peripheral blood of patients with SJS and TEN, and sera from these patients are able to induce marked keratinocyte apoptosis in vitro. It has, thus been proposed that sFasL levels may be an early marker for these two diseases. In addition to soluble factors, there is some evidence that keratinocyte cell death may be mediated directly by cytotoxic T cells since lymphocyte isolated from the blister fluid of a patient with TEN were cytotoxic towards autologous cells only in the presence of the precipitating drug. The apoptotic mechanism appeared to be mediated by perforin/granzyme. [6]

Drugs most commonly implicated	**Drugs occasionally implicated**
Allopurinol	Busulfan
Barbiturates	Cephalosporins
Carbamazepine	Chlorpropamide
NSAIDs	Clindamycin
Penicillin	Codeine
Phenytoin	Ethambutol
Sulfonamides	Furosemide

4) DRUG INDUCED LINEAR Ig A DISEASE:

Etiopathogenesis:

Linear IgA disease has also been referred to as linear IgA bullous dermatosis (LABD) and linear immunoglobulin A dermatosis. However, like the name suggests LABD develops after drug administration. Literature review reveals various drugs that have known to produce LABD, such as vancomycin, diclofenac, lithium, captopril, cyclosporine glibenclamide, interferon-gamma, iodine contrast agent, phenytoin sodium, somatostatin and sulfamethoxazole/ trimethoprim. [7]

5) DRUG-INDUCED MELANOSIS:

Etiopathogenesis:

Medications may induce a variety of different forms of mucocutaneous pigmentation, including melanosis. Pigmentation that is caused by the soft tissue deposition of drug metabolites or complexes and pigment associated with deposition of lipofuscin or iron are discussed later in this chapter. The chief drugs implicated in drug-induced melanosis are the antimalarials, including chloroquine, hydroxyl chloroquine, quinacrine, and others. In the Western world, these medications are typically used for the treatment of autoimmune disease. Other common classes of medications that induce melanosis include the phenothiazines, such as chlorpromazine, oral contraceptives, and cytotoxic medications such as cyclophosphamide and busulfan. [8]

A. INFECTIONS:

1) VIRAL:

i) HERPES SIMPLEX VIRUS:

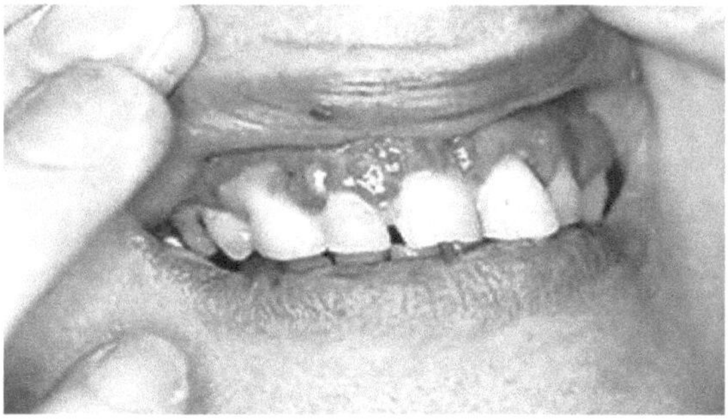

Fig 1: Primary herpes simplex of gingiva in an adult. [8]

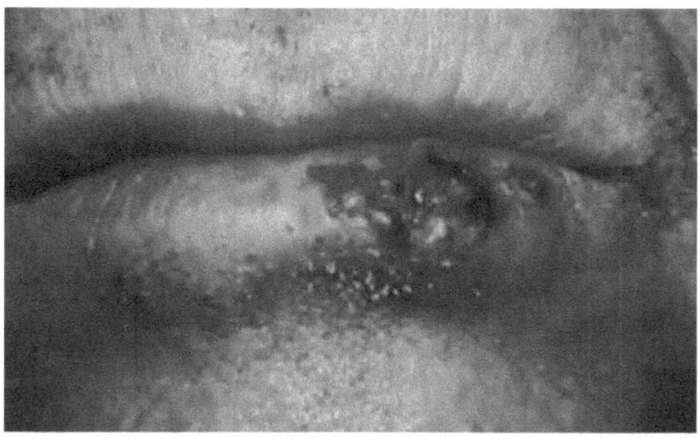

Fig 2: Crusted lesions of recurrent herpes labialis. [8]

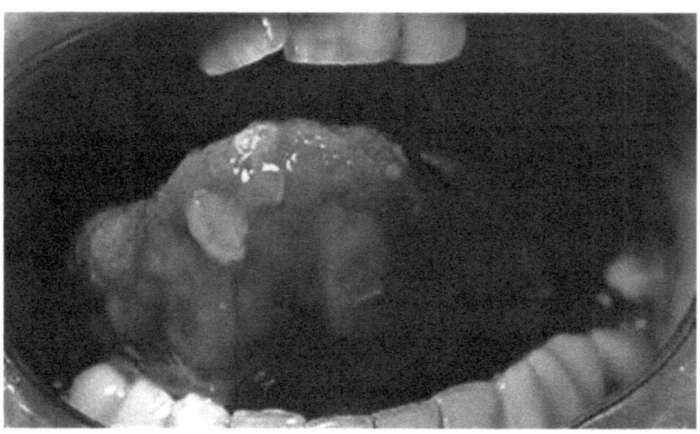

Fig 3: Herpes simplex of the tongue. [8]

Clinical features:

Affected patients present with acute onset of multiple vesicles and ulcerations, inflamed gingiva, cervical Iymphadenopathy, and an elevated temperature. Discomfort is often severe, inhibiting normal ingestion of food and liquids. As a result, dehydration may occur, necessitating fluid replacement therapy. Occasionally, primary herpetic gingivostomatitis occurs in adults who are exposed to the virus for the first time later in life. In these patients, the condition tends to run a more severe clinical course. [10]

ii) VARICELLA ZOSTER VIRUS:

Clinical features:

Prodromal symptoms of pain or paraesthesia develop and persist for several days as the virus infects the sensory nerve of a dermatome (usually of the trunk or head and neck). A vesicular skin eruption that becomes pustular and eventually ulcerated follows. The disease lasts several weeks and may be followed by a troublesome post-herpetic neuralgia (in approximately 15% of patients) that takes several months to resolve. Local cutaneous hyperpigmentation may also be noted on occasion. Cytological examination of the contents of vesicles is carried out for varicella and herpes zoster in the same way as for herpes simplex. It is a very useful diagnostic test, confirming the diagnosis in 80% to 100% of the cases, whereas viral cultures can confirm in only 60% to 64%. [11]. (Refer Fig: 4 and 5)

iii) HAND-FOOT-AND-MOUTH DISEASE:

Clinical features:

Symptoms usually appear 3 to 5 days after exposure. After a 1-to 2-day mild prodrome of low-grade fever, sore throat, and malaise, small red macules present on the oral mucosal and progress to 1- to 3-mm vesicles, where they evolve into small ulcers. Between 25% and 65% of patients may have the classic vesicular lesions on the hand and feet, which presented as scattered small vesicles surrounded by an erythematous halo on the palms of the hands, soles of the feet, and ventral surfaces and sides of the fingers and toes. Similar lesions may develop on the rest of the skin. [11] (Refer Fig: 6)

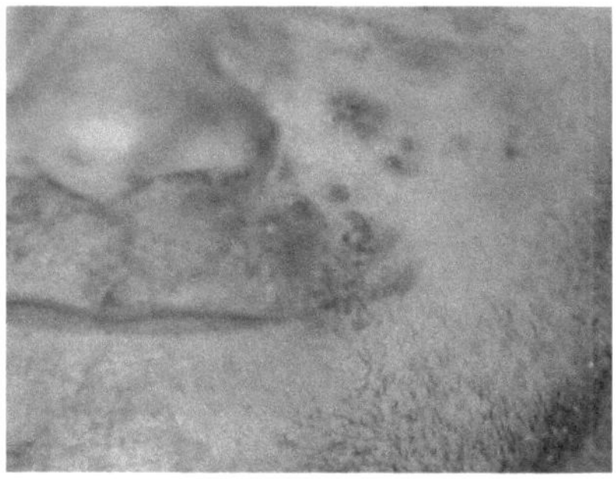

Fig 4: Facial lesions of varicella zoster involving the trigeminal nerve. [8]

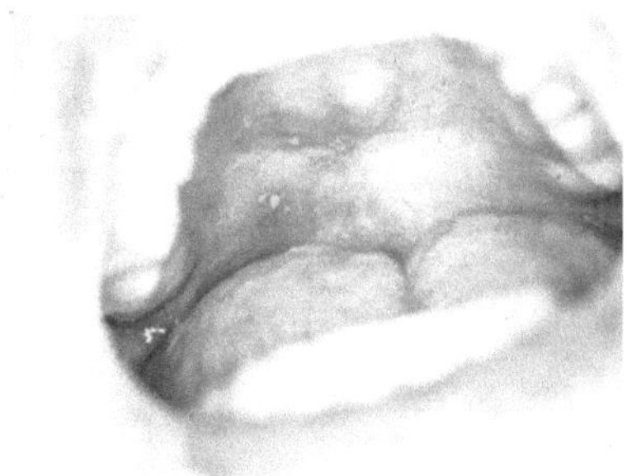

Fig 5: Palatal lesions of varicella zoster of second division of the trigeminal nerve. [8]

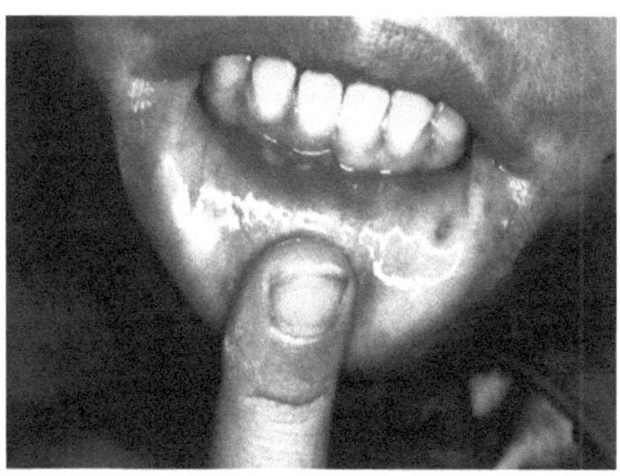

Fig 6: Eruption of small vesicles on lower lip. [16]

iv) HERPANGINA:

Clinical features:

It is more common in children than in adults. Those infected generally complain of malaise, fever, dysphagia, and sore throat after a short incubation period. Intraorally a vesicular eruption appears on the soft palate, faucial pillars, and tonsils. A diffuse erythematous pharyngitis is also present. The signs and symptoms are usually mild to moderate and generally last less than a week. Diagnosis is usually based on historical and clinical information. The characteristic distribution and short duration of herpangina separate it from other primary viral infections such as herpetic gingivostomatitis and varicella. The vesicular eruption, mild symptoms, summer or early autumn presentation, and diffuse pharyngitis also distinguish the condition from streptococcal pharyngitis, and the systemic symptoms distinguish it from aphthous stomatitis. [11]. (Refer Fig: 7)

2) BACTERIAL:

i) IMPETIGO:

Clinical features:

When the condition disseminates to affect various parts of the body, it is referred to as staphylococcal scalded skin syndrome. This is usually seen in immunocompromised patients. The toxin may disseminate hematogenously and lead to generalized staphylococcal scalded skin syndrome. Bullous impetigo can affect any part of the skin and mucosa. Literature review reveals few reports of buccal mucosa involvement. The initial lesion appears as small to large, superficial, fragile bullae. These bullae usually occur on the extremities, axille and the trunk. Some patients report history of trauma or infections. These bullae are generally painless. However some patients experience burning or itching sensation. The bullae measure about 2 to 5 cm in size and usually do not rupture easily. They contain a serous clear yellow fluid that subsequently turns cloudy and dark yellow. In about 3–4 days time the bullae rupture and produce a thin, light brown, varnish-like or honey like crust. A characteristic finding in bullous impetigo is a 'collarette' of scale surrounding the blister roof at the periphery of ruptured lesions. [7] (Refer Fig: 8)

ii) GONORRHOEA

Clinical Features:

Infection in males results in acute urethritis, dysuria and urethral discharge of a purulent nature. Some patients may have mucoid discharge. It may lead to epididymitis, chronic prostatitis, balanitis and posterior urethritis. In females, it manifests as cervicitis with candidal or trichomonal vaginitis. Mostly they are symptomatic. Carrier symptoms include vaginal discharge, discomfort, and dysuria. It may affect the rectum, oropharynx, and the eye. [1]

Oral Manifestations:

Extragenital gonorrheal infection of oral cavity is being seen with increasing frequency, especially among but not confined to homosexuals, and occurs as a result of oral-genital contact or inoculation through infected hands. Transmission by fomites is rare. Schmidt and coworkers have reviewed the literature on gonococcal stomatitis and have pointed out the clinical similarity between the oral lesions of this disease and the oral lesions of erythema multiforme, erosive or bullous lichen planus, and herpetic stomatitis. Chue has also reviewed this disease, describing the various oral lesions in detail. The lips may develop acute painful ulceration, limiting motion; the gingiva may become erythe-matous, with or without necrosis; and the tongue may present red, dry ulcerations or become glazed and swollen with painful erosions, with similar lesions on the buccal mucosa and palate. Gonococcal pharyngitis and tonsillitis are also well recognized lesions. These appear as vesicles or ulcers with a grey or white pseudomembrane. Oral lesions are commonly accompanied by fever and regional lymphadenopathy. Finally, gonococcal parotitis, presumably a result of an ascending infection from the duct to the gland, has been reported on numerous occasions. [1]. Refer Fig: 9.

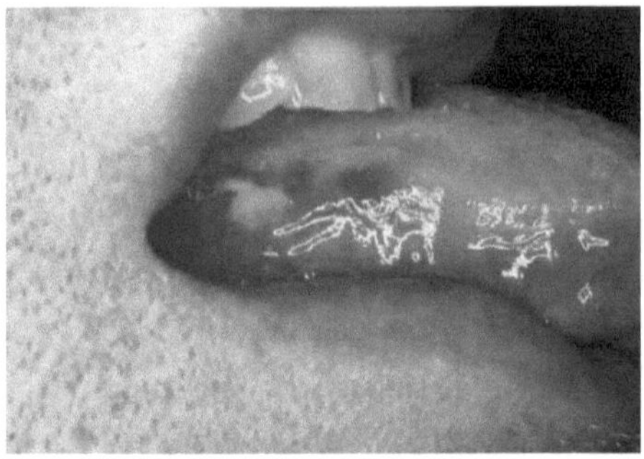

Fig 7: A cluster of ulcers on the tongue of a patient with herpangina. [8]

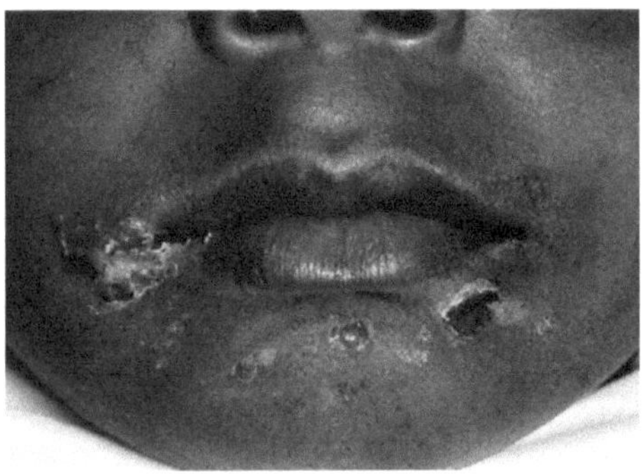

Fig 8: Impetigo. Pustular and crusted perioral lesions commonly harboring Streptococcus pyogenes and Staphylococcus aureus pathogens in a young patient. [16]

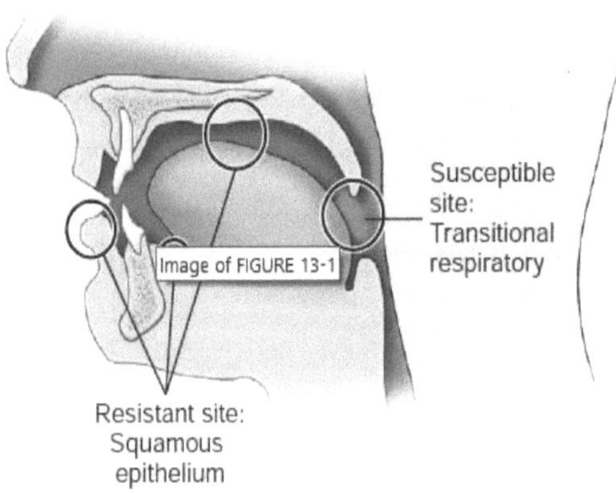

Fig 9: Areas of relative epithelial susceptibility to infection by Neisseria gonorrhoeae within the oral cavity. [17]

iii) CAT SCRATCH DISEASE:

Clinical Features:

This disease, occurring at any age, but predominantly in children and young adults, is thought to arise after a traumatic break in the skin due to the scratch or bite of the household cat. On rare occasions, dogs and monkeys have served as the vector. Actually, there is a definite history of scratches in only 55–60% of patients, according to Rickles and Bernier, although 90% of patients with the disease had recent contact with cats. The primary lesion is often a papule, pustule or vesicle that develops at the site of the injury. Within one to three weeks, a regional lymphadenitis without lymphangitis develops. The cat apparently serves only as a carrier of the disease, since the animal is not ill and does not respond to the intradermal antigen test. The lymphadenopathy is usually the cause for the patients seeking professional advice. In a series of 115 patients with clinical cat-scratch disease reported by Margileth, 57% had lymphadenopathy involving the extremities, and 43%, the head and neck. The nodes are painful and may be several centimeters in diameter. The overlying skin may be inflamed. This lymphadenopathy may persist for one to six months and may be accompanied in the early stages of the disease by a low-grade fever, headache, chills, nausea, malaise, or even abdominal pain. Other manifestations occasionally seen include a nonpruritic macular or maculopapular rash, parotid swelling, conjunctivitis, and grand mal seizures. Another unusual manifestation of the disease, reported by Carithers, is the oculoglandular syndrome of Parinaud. This consists of a localized granuloma of the eye and preauricular lymphadenopathy. The lymph nodes gradually become soft and fluctuant, owing to necrosis and suppuration. Pus has been reported in numerous studies to be bacteriologically sterile. Occasionally, an abscessed node will perforate the skin and drain. If the preauricular, submaxillary, or cervical chain of nodes are involved, the dentist may be consulted to rule out dental disease as an etiologic factor. Cat-scratch disease may also resemble more serious infectious granulomatous diseases such as tuberculosis or tularemia, lymphogranuloma venereum, infectious mononucleosis, or Hodgkin's disease and lymphosarcoma. [1]

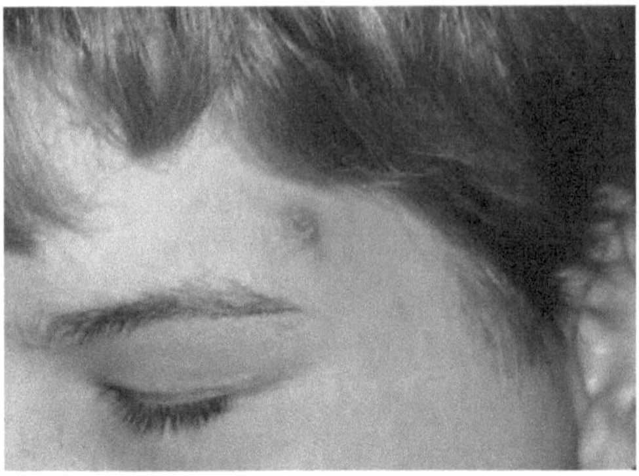

Fig 10: Cat-scratch disease. Papule that developed at initial site of injury. [18]

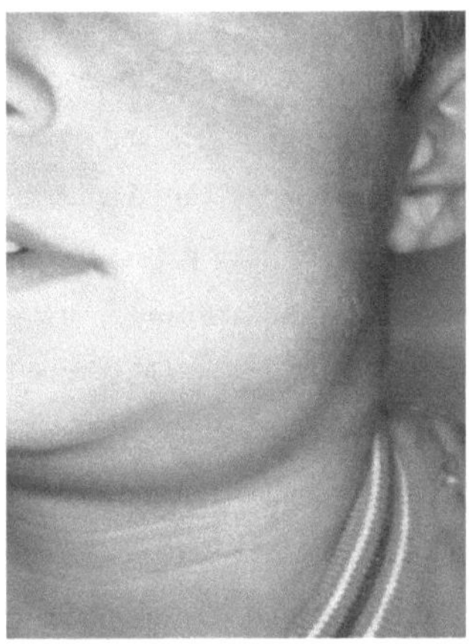

Fig 11: Cat-scratch disease. Submandibular lymphadenopathy has developed after initial trivial injury to skin. [18]

3) FUNGAL:

Clinical Features:

Blastomycosis is typically seen in men engaged in outdoor activities usually in the 3rd and 4th decades of life. The acute form of blastomycosis is characterized by fever, malaise, myalgias, weight loss, cough, and pleuritic chest pain. The chronic form is much more commonly seen than the acute form. It is characterized by symptoms mimicking those of tuberculosis such as night sweats, low-grade fever, productive cough and weight loss. Rarely, dissemination to other body sites such as the skin, bone, CNS, genitourinary system and oral cavity may be seen. Cutaneous lesions may appear as erythematous nodules that subsequently ulcerate. [7] (Refer Fig: 12)

Oral features:

Intraoral lesions of blastomycosis appear as irregular pink or white areas. The ulcers may be painful and appear irregular with rolled borders. [7].

4) CHLAMYDEAL:

Clinical Features:

Groove sign: Originally described by Greenblatt in lymphogranuloma venereum (LGV). Enlargement of lymph nodes above and below the inguinal ligament may give to bubo a grooved appearance known as groove sign. [19]

Oral Considerations:

Orogenital contact may result in the primary lesion of lymphogranuloma venereum occurring in the mouth. The tongue is the most frequently affected site in primary infections, and the lesion appears as a painless vesicle. As the disease progresses, the tongue may become enlarged, with areas of scarring and deep grooves on the dorsum. The grooves are intensely red, with loss of superficial epithelium, or, alternatively, grayish opaque papules may develop. Other areas of the mouth may be involved, and lesions of the lips, cheeks, tongue, floor of the mouth, uvula, and pharynx have been described. The cervical lymph nodes become painfully enlarged within 7 days to 2 months after the appearance of the initial lesions and may suppurate, forming abscesses and fistulae. [8]. (Refer Fig: 13)

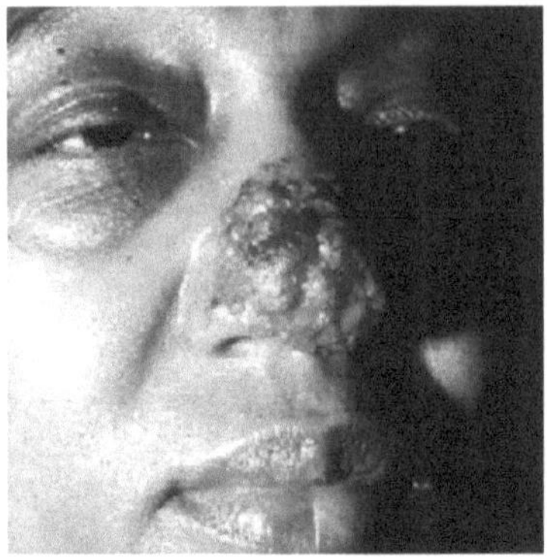

Fig 12: Blastomycosis, dissemination to the nose. [16]

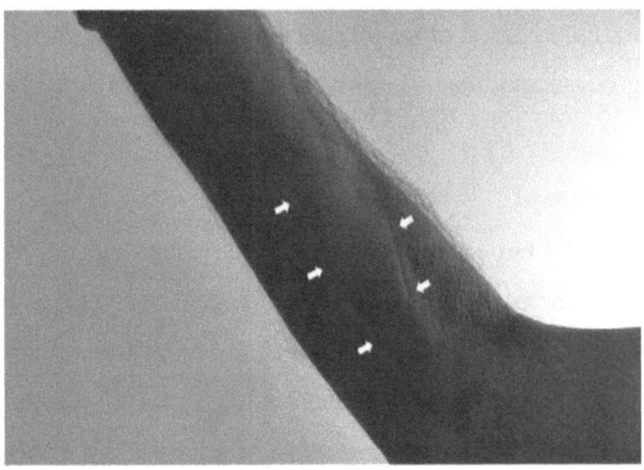

Fig 13: Right arm of the patient elevated. Groove sign: The grooves on the skin of the inner forearm (white arrows) are seen. [19]

B) SKIN DISEASES:

1. PEMPHIGUS VULGARIS:

Clinical features:

PV affects the mucosa and the skin, resulting in superficial blisters and chronic ulcerations. Various mucosal surfaces may be involved, including ocular, nasal, oral, pharangeal, laryngeal, upper respiratory, and anogenital mucous membranes. Classic lesion is flaccid thin walled bullae that may arise on normal or erythematous skin/mucous membrane. The bulla are fragile & break readily leaving denuded areas of variable size that tend to enlarge as the epithelium detaches from the dermis at the periphery. Such vesicles and bullae rupture easily on the skin, so that the most common skin lesions seen are erosions, which may be widespread. Skin lesions consists of WEEPING bulla that bursts, crusts and recur in the same area and spread to adjacent regions. The formation of a lesion after gentle mechanical pressure (blowing air / applying pressure with mirror handle) on affected tissue may be used as a diagnostic tool in the assessment of patients presenting with oral ulcerations. This test is known as NIKOLSKY'S SIGN, named after Pyotr Vasilyewich nikolsky, who first described this sign (may also be seen in MMP, Epidermolysis bullosa). [12]

ASBOC-HANSEN SIGN: When finger is applied directly over an intact blister it produces lateral spread of lesion. [12]

Oral manifestations:

80-90% of patients with pemphigus vulgaris develop oral lesions sometime during the course of disease, and, in 60% of cases, the oral lesions are the first sign. Oral lesions usually begins as a vesicle or bulla. Early oral lesions may consist of a single hemorrhagic bulla or shallow ill-defined irregular ulcers. However a whitish superficial covering which is the collapsed roof of a bulla is consistent and characteristic finding. Blisters, which rapidly lead to chronic erosions and ulcers, are seen mainly in the buccal mucosa, palate, ventral surface of tongue and lips. Pemphigus should be considered whenever there are multiple persistent oral erosions, but in the early stages, the erosions may be recurrent. Advanced signs usually consist of severe desquamative or erosive gingivitis, but gingival lesions are uncommon at the onset or may appear as isolated blister or erosions, or both, mainly on free gingiva, and may be difficult to recognize as bullous lesions. Lips may be covered by thick hemorrhagic crusts. In advanced cases, the lesions may resemble ERYTHEMA MULTIFORME. Gentle lateral pressure applied to an area adjacent to the affected site forms a blister resulting in a positive nikolsky's sign. Distal extension from oral cavity can occur effecting oesophagus, pharynx, larynx producing dysphagia and odynophagia. In the present case flaccid fluid filled bullae was seen on the lower lip and a positive nikolsky's sign was also elicited. Areas of desquamation involving the marginal and attached gingival which showed bleeding on probing were also seen. The oral lesions were the only presenting symptoms without skin or any other mucosal involvement. [12]. (Refer Fig 14, 15, 16 and 17)

2) BULLOUS PEMPHIGOID:

Clinical Features:

Oral lesions begin as bullae, but they tend to rupture sooner, probably as a result of constant low-grade trauma to which the oral mucosa is subjected. Large, shallow ulcerations with smooth, distinct margins are present after the bullae rupture. Sometimes erosions are confined to the gingiva creating a picture of chronic desquamative gingivitis. [13]. (Refer Fig 18 and 19)

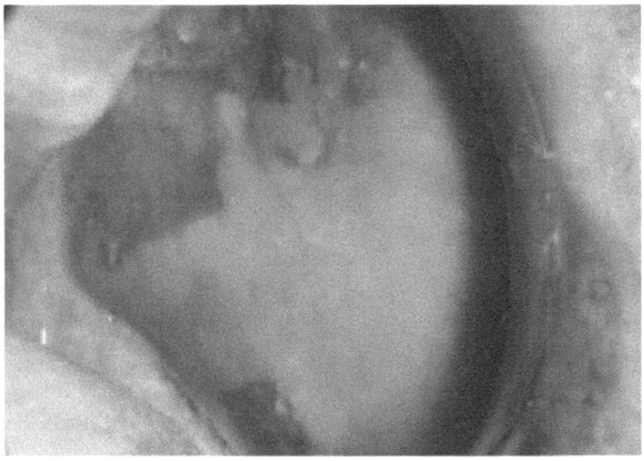

Fig 14: Pemphigus vulgaris. Multiple erosions of the left buccal mucosa. [18]

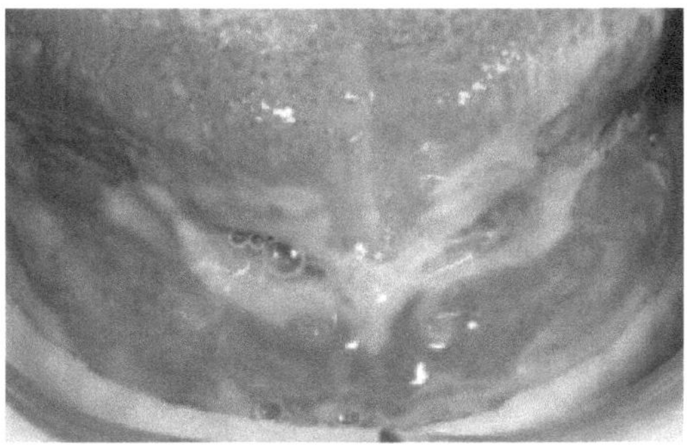

Fig 15: Pemphigus vulgaris. Large, irregularly shaped ulceration involving the floor of the mouth and ventral tongue. [18]

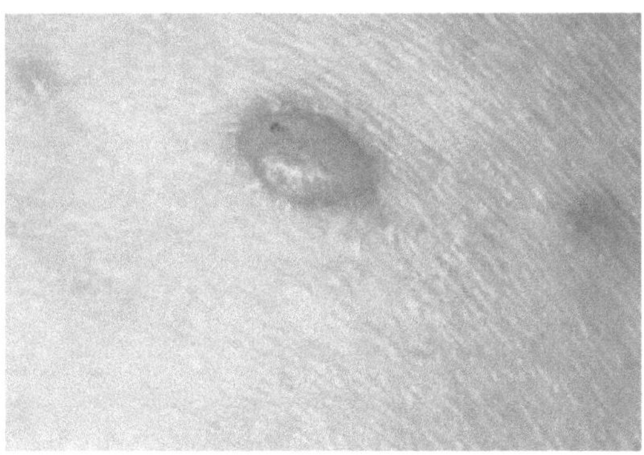

Fig 16: Pemphigus vulgaris. This flaccid cutaneous bulla is characteristic of skin involvement. [18]

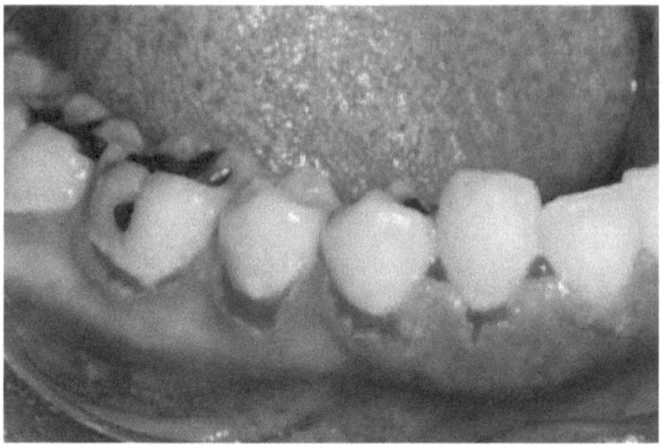

Fig 17: Pemphigus vulgaris. Multiple erosions affecting the marginal gingiva. [18]

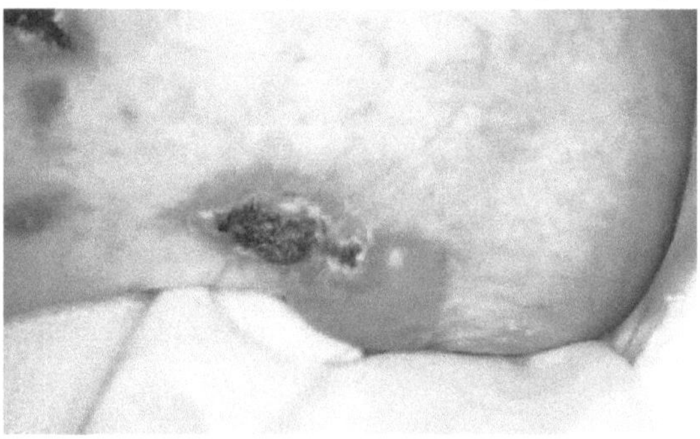

Fig 18: Bullous pemphigoid. Cutaneous vesiculobullous lesions of the heel. The bullae eventually rupture, leaving hemorrhagic crusted areas. [18]

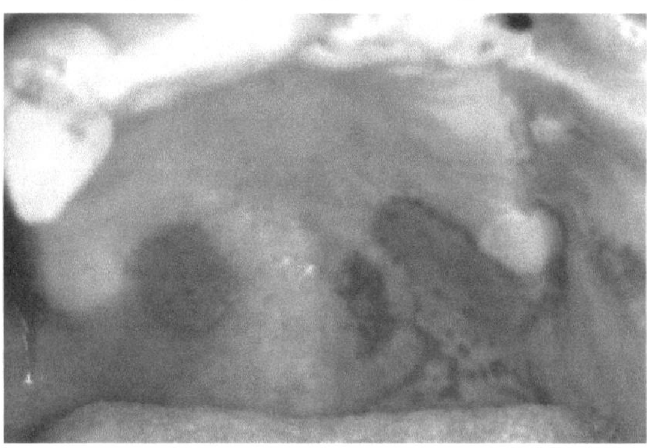

Fig 19: Bullous pemphigoid. These oral lesions appear as large, shallow ulcerations involving the soft palate. [18]

3) MUCOUS MEMBRANE PEMPHIGOID:

Clinical Features:

Oral MMP usually appears suddenly, is painful, waxes and wanes in severity and lasts for years or may be active throughout the remainder of the patient's life. Oral lesions are not life threatening, but may be associated with considerable morbidity in severely affected patients who do not respond to medication. The attending dentist must always rule out ocular and respiratory tract lesions. Patients who respond to treatment usually require constant or at least intermittent therapy for years. [14]. (Refer Fig 20, 21 and 22)

4) LUPUS ERYTHEMATOSUS:

Clinical Features:

Oral lesions of SLE develop in 5% to 25% of patients. The lesions usually affect the palate, buccal mucosa and gingiva. Sometimes they appear as lichenoid areas, but they may also look nonspecific or even somewhat granulomatous. Involvement of the vermilion zone of the lower lip (lupus cheilitis) is sometimes seen. Varying degrees of ulceration, pain, erythema and hyperkeratosis may be present. Other oral complaints are xerostomia, stomatodynia, candidiasis, periodontal disease and dysgeusia. Oral or nasopharyngeal ulceration is recognized as a major diagnostic manifestation of SLE by the American Rheumatism Association Committee on Diagnostic and Therapeutic Criteria. These ulcerations are generally painless and often involve the palate. Purpuric lesions such as ecchymoses and petechiae may also occur. [13]. (Refer Fig: 23)

5) DERMATITIS HERPETIFORMIS:

Clinical Features:

Periods of exacerbation and remission further characterize this disease. Lesions are usually symmetric in their distribution over the extensor surfaces, especially the elbows, shoulders, sacrum, and buttocks. Of diagnostic significance is the frequent involvement of the scalp and face. Lesions are usually aggregated (herpetiformis) but often are individually disposed. In the oral cavity, dermatitis herpetiformis is very rare, with vesicles and bullae having been described that rupture, leaving superficial nonspecific ulcers with a fibrinous base with erythematous margins. Lesions may involve both keratinized and nonkeratinized mucosa. [12]. (Refer Fig: 24)

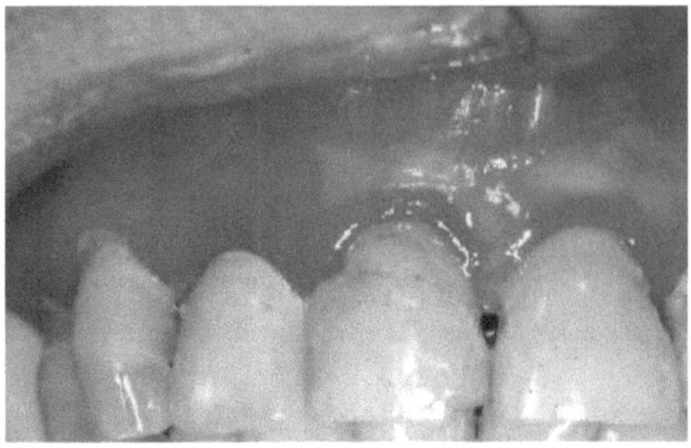

Fig 20: Chronic desquamative gingival lesions of mucous membrane pemphigoid. [8]

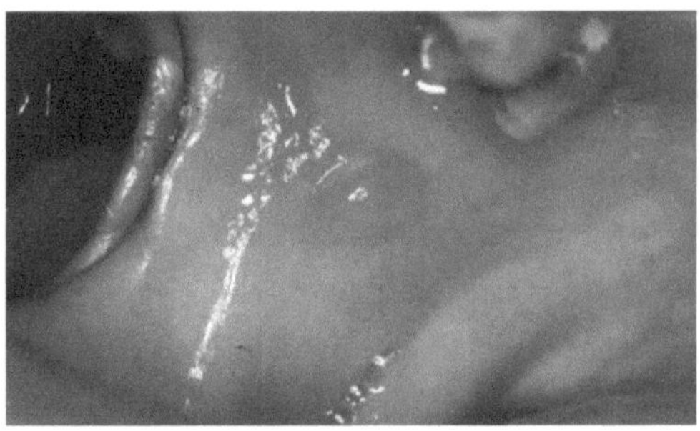

Fig 21: Intact vesicle of buccal mucosa with mucous membrane pemphigoid. [8]

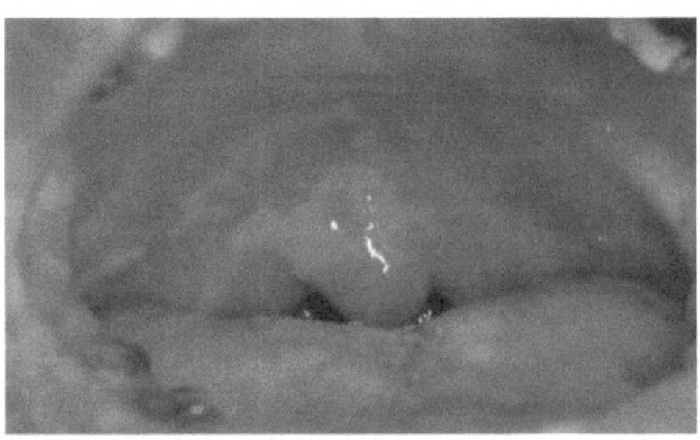

Fig 22: Mucous membrane pemphigoid causing lesions of the soft palate. [8]

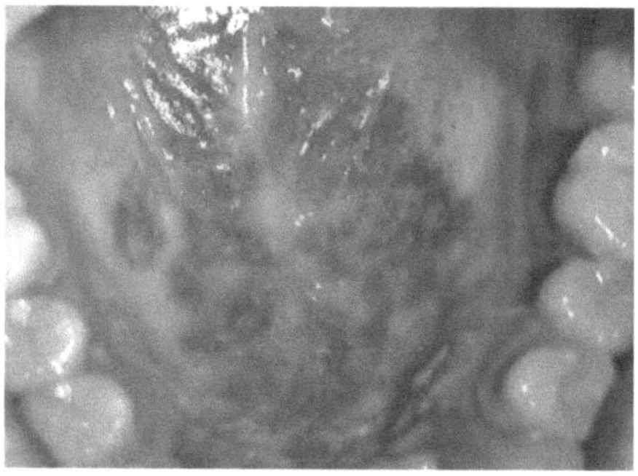

Fig 23: Lupus lesion in the palatal mucosa in a patient with systemic lupus erythematosus. [8]

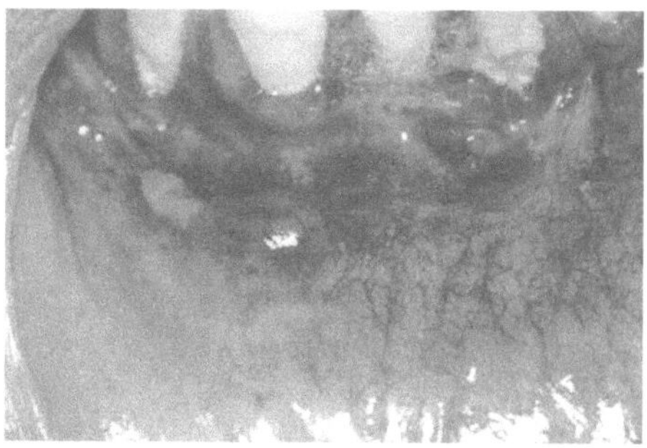

Fig 24: Dermatitis herpetiformis: intact bulla on the lower lip mucosa and small erosions on the gingiva. [20]

6. ORAL LICHEN PLANUS:

Clinical Features:

Oral Mucosal Lichen Planus: [15]

There are majorly 6 forms of Oral Lichen planus:

1)	Reticular	(1) Buccal mucosa and mucobuccal folds. (2) Lateral and dorsal tongue. (3) Gingiva and lips.
2)	Atrophic	Attached gingiva.
3)	Hypertrophic	Buccal mucosa.
4)	Erosive	(1) Lateral and ventral portions of tongue. (2) Buccal mucosa.
5)	Bullous	Posterior and inferior areas of buccal mucosa.
6)	Plaque-like	Dorsum of the tongue and buccal mucosa.

Mucosal LP more commonly involves the oral mucosa but can also affect the vulvovaginal area. LP can rarelymanifest in the esophagus, larynx, and conjunctiva. OLP has several clinical subtypes including reticular, erosive, atrophic, papular, plaque-like, and bullous subtypes.The buccal mucosa is typically involved in 80–90% of OLP cases. The Koebner phenomenon is not only present in CLP but can also occur in the setting of OLP. Eisen suggested that the mechanical trauma of dental procedures, cigarette smoking, mucosal trauma from sharp cusps, and oral habits such as lip chewing are Koebnerogenic factors that can exacerbate OLP. Reticular OLP, the most common subtype, is usually asymptomatic. Hence, it is often diagnosed during a routine oral examination. Reticular OLP is characterized by white lacy streaks surrounded by well-defined erythematous borders. This pattern is less evident on the dorsum of the tongue. In some patients, reticular OLP may eventually progress tothemore severe subtypes such as the erosive form. Papular OLP is characterized by small white pinpoint Papules that can be easily missed as they are small and asymptomatic. It is referred to as the initial and transient phase of OLP. That is why it is a rare diagnosis. In plaque-like OLP, large, homogenous white patches are characteristic. Plaque like OLP and leukoplakia have similar clinical presentations and therefore leukoplakia must always be ruled out. This variant is more prevalent in tobacco smokers. The existence of plaque-like lesions is an indicator of a poor prognosis and a lesser likelihood of remission. Erosive OLP, the most advanced subtype, can clinically present as atrophic or erythematous ulcerations and erosions of the mucosa and faint radiating white striae. The associated ulcers are sometimes covered with a pseudomembrane. Typically, it has a multifocal pattern of distribution. It is clinically important because the lesions can be quite painful and therefore it may negatively affect the patient's quality of life. The symptoms may range from discomfort to severe, painful episodes. Involvement of the dorsum of the tongue might cause dysgeusia. The atrophic subtype is common presentation that has similarities to the erosive subtype with more prominent atrophic lesions on a background of erythema and radiating white striae at the margins. Thus, some experts combine the two entities and name it atrophicerosive lichen planus. This subtype is more common in older OLP patients. Atrophic OLP primarily affects the attached gingiva. The buccal mucosa can also be involved, particularly in the posteroinferior areas adjacent to the second and third molar teeth. In rare instances, OLP may present with bullous lesions. Lourenc¸o and colleagues suggested a rare form of OLP as "Lichen planus sialadenitis," amucosal analog of LPP due to lymphocyte infiltration in the salivary gland ducts. [15]

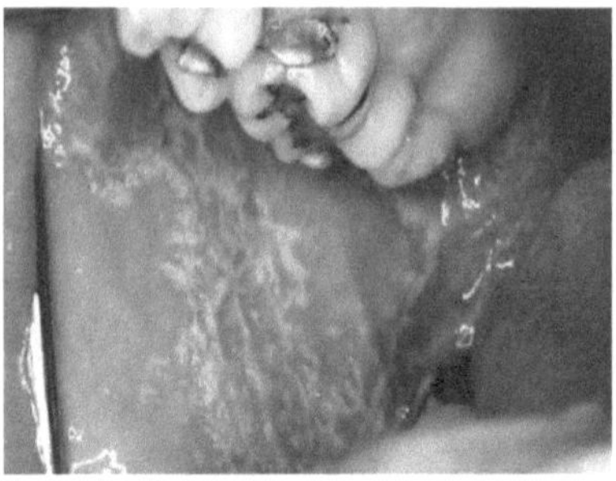

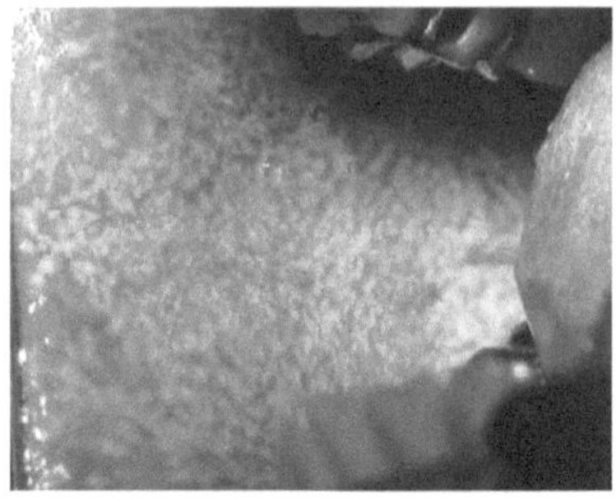

Fig 25: A reticular form. [8].

Fig 26: Papular form [8].

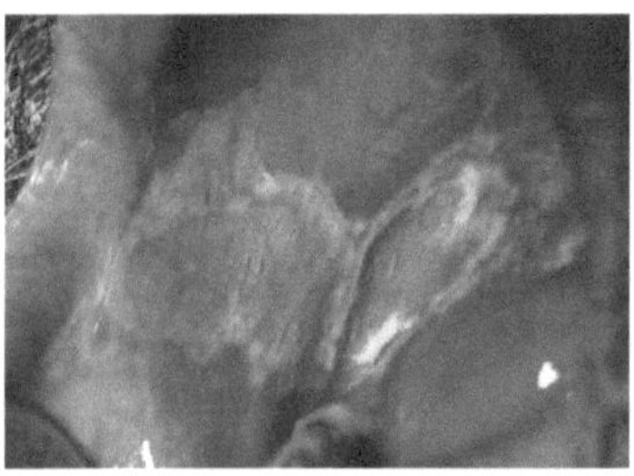

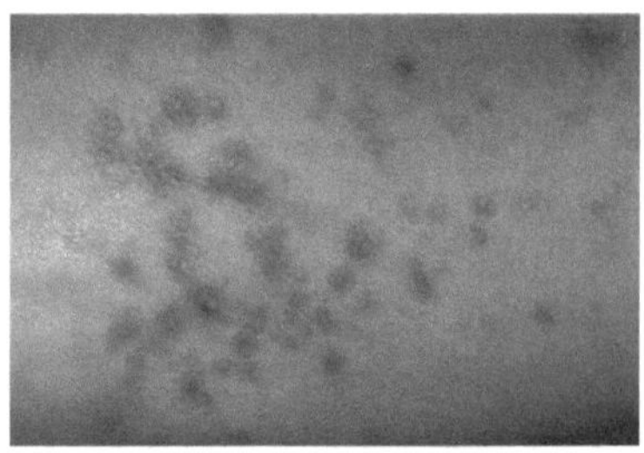

Fig 27: A plaque – like form. [8]

Fig 31: Cutaneous lichen planus. [8].

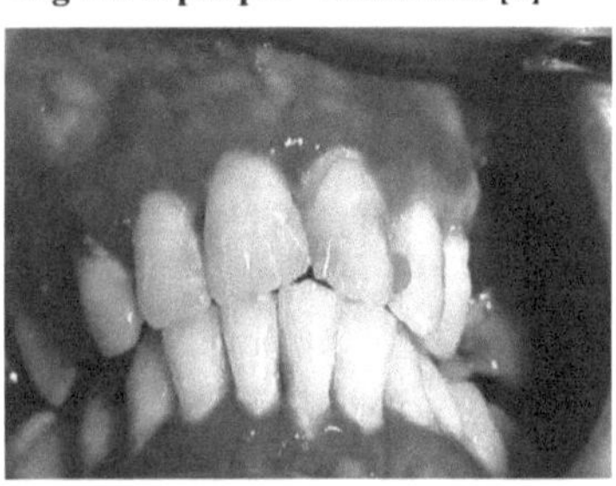

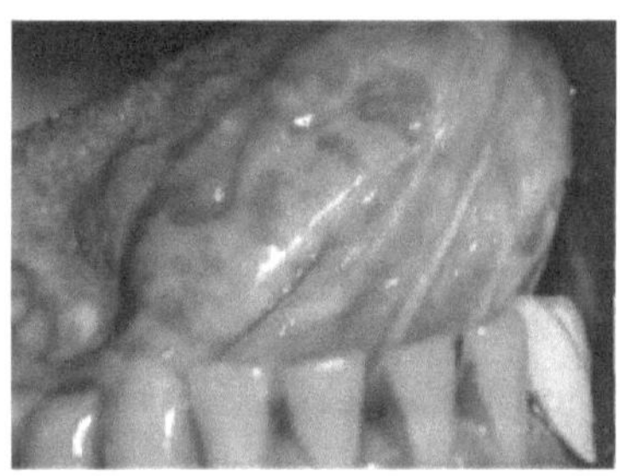

Fig 28: Erythematous oral lichen planus.

Fig 29: Ulcerative oral lichen planus.

[8]

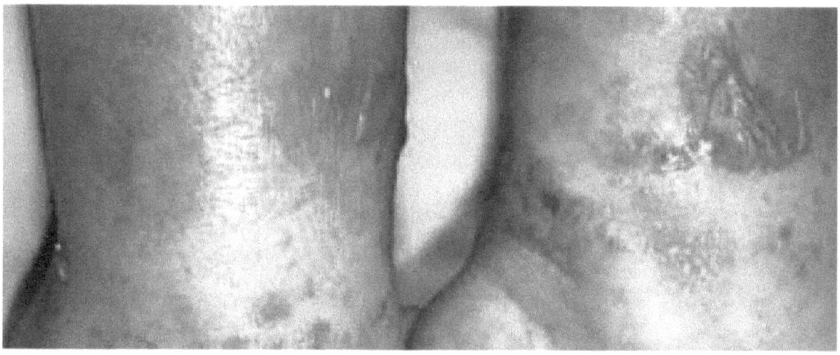

Fig 30: Bullous lichen planus. [15]

7) ERYTHEMA MULTIFORME:

Clinical Features:

Erythema multiforme may present a wide spectrum of severity, from mild limited disease to a severe, widespread and life-threatening illness. Skin lesions are usually symmetrical and consist of macules or erythematous papules, which develop into classical target or iris lesions. Occasionally, bullae may be seen. Skin lesions are often accompanied by ulceration of mucous membranes particularly the oral cavity. Head and neck manifestations were present in 4 of 79 patients (5%) with EM and 26 of 28 patients (93%) with SJS in one series. In SJS, mucosal involvement of the lip (93%), conjunctiva (82%), oral cavity (79%) and nose (36%) were most common. Most patients with EM (70%) of either minor or major forms have oral lesions (Fig. 11.3). Oral involvement may precede lesions on other stratified squamous epithelia, or may arise in isolation. It typically presents with;

• Lesions that progress through diffuse and widespread macules to blisters and ulceration

• Lips that become swollen and cracked, bleeding and get crusted.

• Intraoral lesions typically on the nonkeratinized mucosae and most pronounced in the anterior parts of the mouth.

Recurrences are seen in about 25%; the periodicity can vary from weeks to years; usually attacks last for 10–20 days once or twice a year and usually resolve after about 6 episodes (range: 2–24) within a mean period of 10 years (range: 2–36 years). Skin lesions Skin lesions have been classified as:

1. Typical targets:

They are defined as individual lesions less than 3 cm diameter with a regular round shape, a well-defined border, and two concentric palpable, edematous rings, paler than the center disc. These lesions are most common in EM minor and milder forms of EM major in a symmetrical distribution on the extensor surfaces of the extremities.

2. Raised atypical targets:

It appears similar to target lesions and are palpable erythematous lesions with a rounded shape but poorly defined borders and a dark central area, which may erode and become necrotic. These lesions are most common in severe EM major or in SJS.

3. Flat atypical targets:

As their name suggests are not palpable and they form ill-defined erythematous areas with a tendency to central blister formation. These lesions are most common in SJS.

4. Erythematous or purpuric macules with or without blister formation:

They are of variable size and may become confluent. These lesions are most common in SJS and TEN. Other mucosae

- Eye involvement may cause lacrimation and photophobia.
- Genital lesions are painful and may result in urinary retention. [6]. (Refer Fig: 32 and 33)

8) TOXIC EPIDERMAL NECROLYSIS (TEN):

Clinical Features:

No specific treatment is available but supportive care is important; a liquid diet and intravenous fluid therapy may be necessary. Early ophthalmological and dermatological consultation is needed for diagnosis and management. Precipitating factors, when identified, should be treated. Antimicrobials may be indicated, acyclovir in EM or tetracycline in EM related to M. pneumoniae. A 5-day course of acyclovir at the first sign of lesions, or 400 mg qds for 6 months is useful for prophylaxis in EM. Continuous therapy of valacyclovir, 500 mg twice a day, has also been reported to be effective. The use of corticosteroids is controversial. Minor EM may respond to topical corticosteroids, though systemic corticosteroids may be required and patients with major EM or SJS may need to be admitted for hospital care and should be treated with systemic corticosteroids (prednisolone 0.5–1.0 mg/kg)/day) tapered over 7–10 days) and/or azathioprine or other immunomodulatory drugs. 50% of SJS patients in one series required supplemental hydration or alimentation because of the severity of the oral cavity involvement. Other treatments used, may include cyclophosphamide, dapsone, cyclosporine, azathioprine, levamisole and thalidomide. Plasmapheresis possibly has a place in the management of severe disease. Oral antacids may be helpful for management of discrete oral ulcers. Electrolytes and nutritional support should be started as soon as possible. Oral hygiene should be improved with 0.2% aqueous chlorhexidine mouthwash. [6]. (Refer Fig: 34)

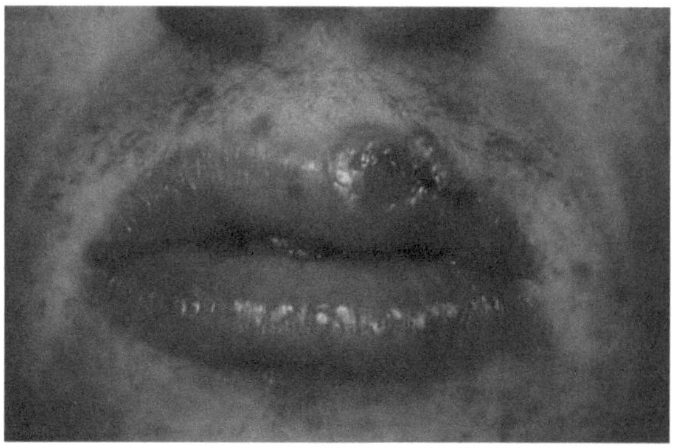

Fig 32: Early vesicular lesions in a patient who develops erythema multiforme after each episode of recurrent herpes labialis. [8].

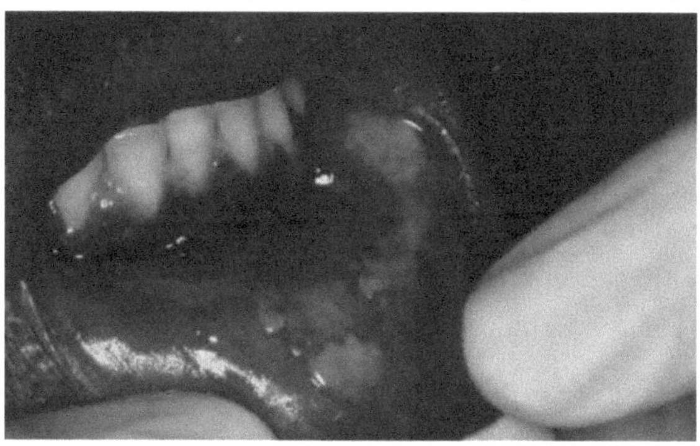

Fig 33: Intraoral lesions of erythema multiforme in an 18-year-old male. [8]

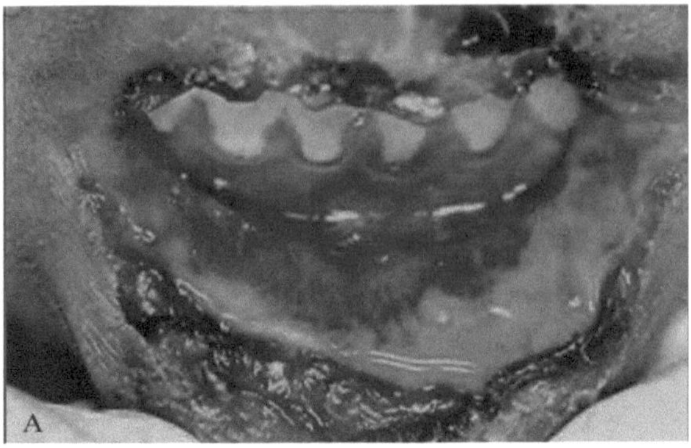

Fig 34: Lips and labial mucosa. [8]

9) EPIDERMOLYSIS BULLOSA:

Clinical Features:

The generalized form of epidermolysis bullosa simplex is inherited as an autosomal dominant characteristic, manifest itself at birth or shortly thereafter and is characterized by the formation of vesicles and bullae, chiefly on the hands and feet at sites of friction or trauma. The knees, elbows and trunk are only occasionally affected. When the blisters heal, usually within 2–10 days, it is an important feature that there is no resultant scarring or permanent pigmentation. The disease appears to improve at puberty and prognosis is good for a normal lifespan. The localized form of the disease (Weber-Cockayne syndrome), which is also familial may occur early in childhood or later in life and is commonly recurrent. The bullae only develop on the hands and feet, are related to frictional trauma and tend to exacerbate in hot weather. There is no scarring upon healing. [6]

Oral Manifestations:

Bullae of the oral cavity have been reported in occasional cases of generalized epidermolysis bullosa simplex, but it is doubtful that they actually occur. In addition, the teeth are not affected. [6]. (Refer Fig: 35)

10) DYSKERATOSIS CONGENITA:

Clinical Features:

Dermatologic Manifestations It occurs in form of reticular hyperpigmentation of skin. These pigmented areas are associated with atrophy of epidermis, capillary hyperplasia and melanin pigment deposited near the blood vessels. Dystrophy of nails is associated with the onset of skin pigmentation. Nail abnormalities can result in longitudinal splitting and furrowing. Nails are brittle or completely lost. In DC eye involvement can lead to epiphora, growth in fundus, blepharitis and loss of eyelashes. Majority of patients develop a hematopoietic disorder resembling Fanconi's anemia because initially the bone marrow is normal but gradually fat cells and fibrotic tissue replace the hematopoietic cells. Hematopoietic disorder manifests as marrow hypoplasia, anemia or thrombocytopenia. With development of pan-cytopenia, there occurs a secondary infection that is the cause of death in majority of these patients. In addition to marrow failure and malignant changes in white patches, pulmonary complications are also serious complications in patients with DC. Immunologic abnormalities occur affecting both the humoral and cell-mediated immunity causing high incidence of opportunistic infections. An abnormality in cell-mediated immunity is evident by delayed hypersensitivity reaction to skin test (antigen inoculation) and no sensitization to dinitrochlorobenzene. Abnormalities in immune systems like lymphoid depletion, absence of primary germinal follicles and fibrosis of lymph nodes can also occur. There may be hyperpigmentation of the buccal mucosa that may be reactive postinflammatory hypermelanosis. Other abnormalities like alopecia, taurodontism, mental retardation, small genitals premature aging, nutmeg liver, horseshoe kidneys, amyloidosis and development of Hodgkin's disease and adenocarcinoma are also reported. [6]

ORAL MANIFESTATIONS:

In DC both the hard and the soft tissues in the oral cavity are affected. Oral mucosal changes manifests in the form of a white keratotic patch. Earlier cases reported of vesicles and ulcerations preceding development of leukoplakia. But these may represent herpetic infections which may occur due to immunocompromised status of these patients secondary to bone marrow suppression. Intraorally, the white patch may affect the buccal mucosa, tongue or palate, with tongue most commonly affected as seen in our patient. Usually, white patch associated with dyskeratosis congenita is leukoplakia but lichen planus or lichenoid lesions instead of leukoplakia are also reported. Lichenoid lesions may be a component of chronic graft-versus-host disease. Electron microscopy studies revealed that cells in dyskeratosis congenita have an embryonic immature nucleus, which have higher chances to undergo malignant transformation. In addition, barrier zone of epithelium is less effective in dyskeratosis congenita than the normal epithelium causing increased permeability of noxious substances and carcinogens to the germinal layers. Hence increased malignant transformation rate is seen in leukoplakic areas associated with dyskeratosis congenita.

In DC severe periodontal destruction occur due to anomalies in ectodermally derived structures and diminished host response caused by neutropenia. Patients have gingival inflammation, bleeding, recession and bone loss that simulates juvenile periodontitis. In addition, there may be defects in the structure of the enamel like hypocalcification that may cause dental caries. [6]. (Refer Fig: 36)

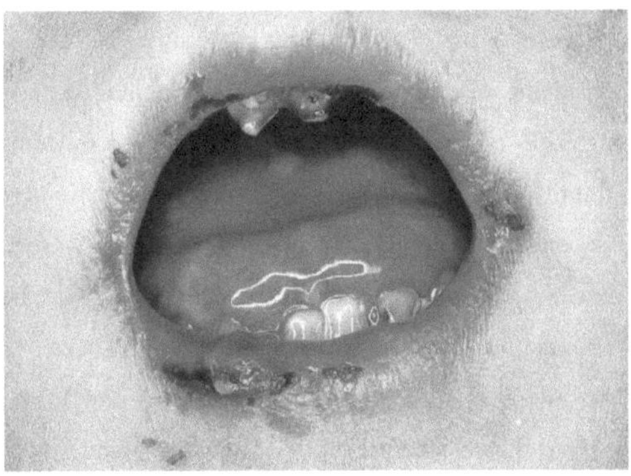

Fig 35: Epidermolysis bullosa in a child. Note ulcers, constricted opening, and atrophic tongue mucosa. [21].

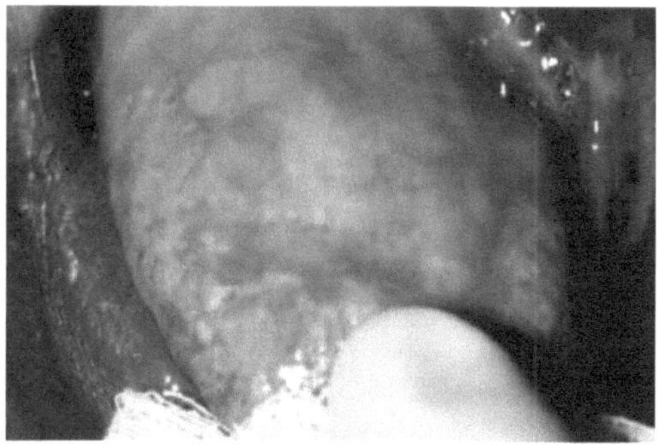

Fig 36: Dyskeratosis congenita. Atrophy and hyperkeratosis of the dorsal tongue mucosa are visible. [18]

C) DRUG INDUCED:

1) LICHENOID REACTION:

Clinical Features:

They are present as reticular, erythematous, erosive lesions or ulcerations, with whitish streak similar to that of Wickham's striae of lichen planus. Clinical manifestations of LR are very much similar to that of lichen planus. An important factor which distinguishes LR from lichen planus is its atypical location and absence of bilateral occurrence. [1]. (Refer Fig: 37)

2) PEMPHIGUS FOLIACEUS:

Clinical Features:

Pemphigus foliaceus is manifested by characteristic early bullous lesions which rapidly rupture and dry to leave masses of flakes or scales suggestive of an exfoliative dermatitis or eczema. The disease may originate in this form or may develop from one of the other types of pemphigus. It is a relatively mild form of pemphigus, which is most common in older adults but may occur in young children as well. [1]. (Refer Fig: 38)

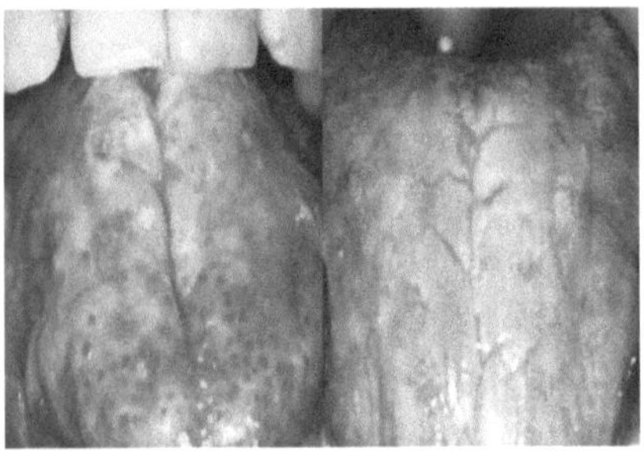

Fig 37: A. Drug-induced lichenoid reaction following 1 month of medication with a cholestyramine - containing drug.
B. Three weeks following withdrawal of the drug. [8]

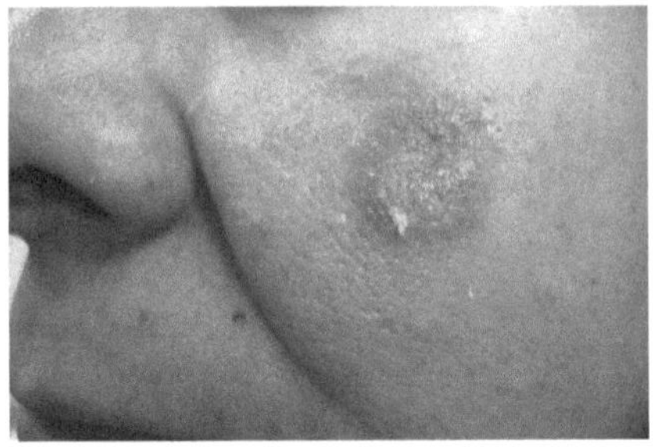

Fig 38: Pemphigus foliaceus. [22]

3) DRUG INDUCED ERYTHEMA MULTIFORME:

Clinical Features:

A wide range of drugs may give rise to EM, and it may be impossible to clinically distinguish drug-induced EM from disease due to other causes. Lesions typically affect the oral mucosa, the lips and bulbar conjunctivae. Initial bullae rupture to give rise to hemorrhagic pseudomembrane of the lips and widespread superficial oral ulceration. Other mucocutaneous surfaces less commonly affected include the nasopharyngeal, respiratory and genital mucosae. [6]. (Refer Fig: 39, 40 and 41)

4) DRUG INDUCED LINEAR IgA disease:

Clinical Features:

Dermal lesions mimic lesions of DH or BP. Vesiculobullous rash may be appreciated over a normal or erythematous dermis. The bullae may contain serous sero-hemorrhagic content. The common sites of involvement include the extensor surfaces of the hand and feet, lower trunk, perioral region, genital region and buttocks. In adults, the trunk and the limbs are usually affected. Lesions may not be symmetric. The bullae may arrange in a herpetiform manner or clusters of discrete bullae, which has been popularly termed as 'jewels sign'. Another characteristic finding is the presence of vesicles or bullae bordering the annular lesion which is termed 'string of beads sign'. Dermal lesions usually heal without scarring. [7]. (Refer Fig: 42)

5) DRUG-INDUCED MELANOSIS:

Clinical Features:

It has been estimated that 10 to 20% of all cases of acquired melanocytic pigmentation may be drug induced. Intraorally, the pigment can be diffuse yet localized to one mucosal surface, often the hard palate, or it can be multifocal and involve multiple surfaces. Some drugs may even be associated with a specific pattern of pigmentation. Much like other forms of diffuse pigmentation, the lesions are flat and without any evidence of nodularity or swelling. Sun exposure may exacerbate cutaneous drug-induced pigmentation. [8]. (Refer Fig: 43)

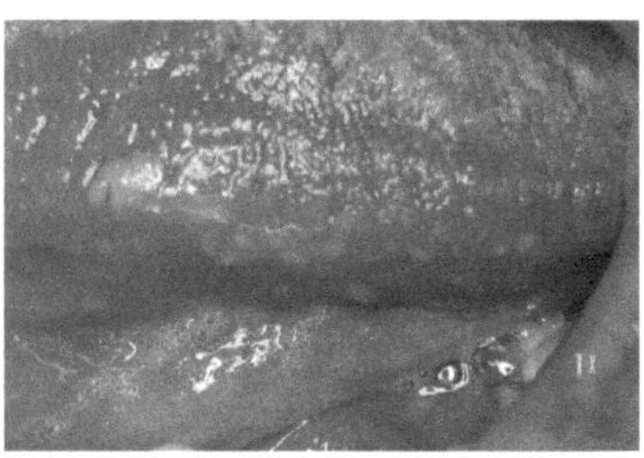

Fig39: A) [21]

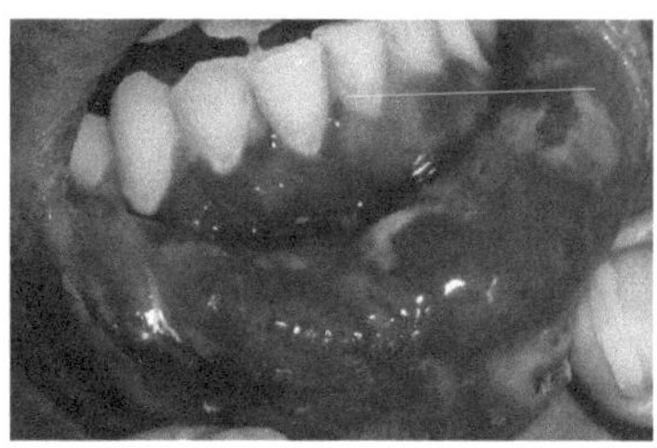

Fig 40: B) [21]

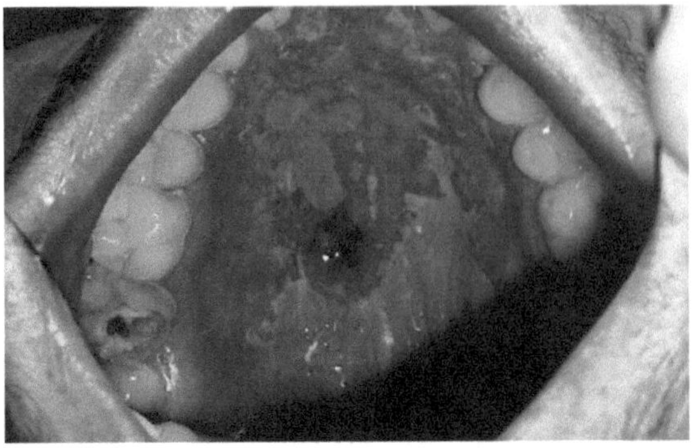

Fig 41: C) Erythema multiforme. A, Erosive lesions of the labial mucosa and gingiva. B, Diffuse area of superficial sloughing and focal erosions of the palate. [16]

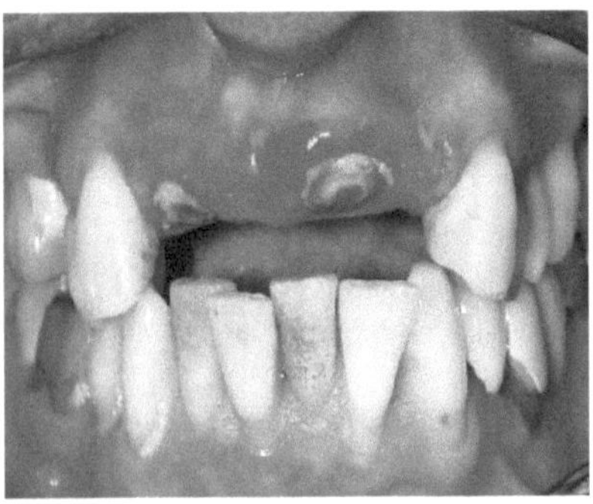

Fig 42: Drug induced linear IgA disease. [23]

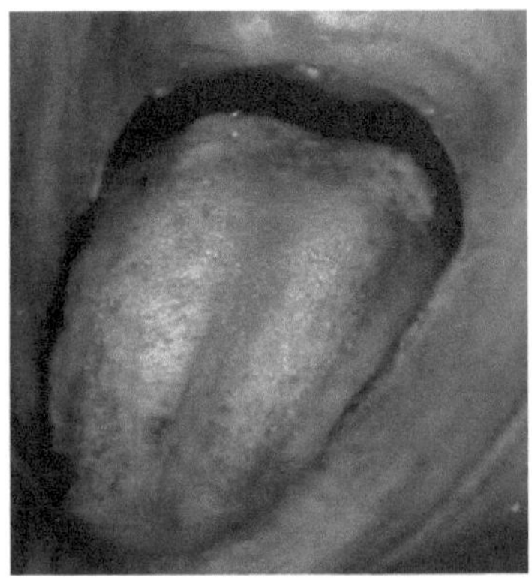

Fig 43: Drug-induced pigmentation of the tongue in a patient who was taking chlorpromazine. [8]

Autoimmune mucocutaneous diseases are generally insidious in onset. They are mainly caused by autoantibodies produced by body's own cells. In the oral cavity these antibodies target the skin components of epithelial cells mainly the basement membrane. Certain human leucocyte antigens of the body's HLA complex is associated with the formation of these autoimmune mucocutaneous diseases. Eg: HLA-DQB1*0301

They include:

1. Mucous membrane pemphigoid
2. Pemphigus vulgaris
3. Pemphigus foliaceus
4. Paraneoplastic pemphigus
5. Bullous pemphigoid
6. Linear Ig A disease
7. Epidermolysis bullosa
8. Oral lichen planus

The symptoms of these diseases are so severe that the patients are prevented from proper dietary intake resulting in severe malnutrition. These diseases can affect any part of oral cavity. The regions include:

1. Gingiva
2. Palate
3. Buccal mucosa
4. Tongue
5. Floor of mouth
6. Pharynx

These diseases follow a neoplastic transformation even. They may be NonHodgkin's Lymphoma, chronic lymphocytic leukemia. [24]

PATHOGENESIS:

Mechanisms hypothesized involved in autoimmune diseases:

1. Failure to delete autoreactive lymphocytes
2. Central tolerance failure
3. Peripheral tolerance failure
4. Molecular mimicry
5. Abnormal presentation of self antigens

6. Aberrant expression of major histocompatibility complex
7. class II molecules
8. Coupling of self and nonself antigens
9. Overproduction of self antigens
10. Disclosure of cryptic T-cell epitopes
11. Release of sequestered self antigens
12. Epitope spreading
13. Polyclonal lymphocyte activation

Failure to delete autoreactive lymphocytes:

The familial association of autoimmune diseases suggests that the aetiopathogenesis of these diseases may be controlled by genetic factors. In certain individuals there might be a genetically determined inability to delete all autoreactive T- and B-cell clones during ontogenesis. Indeed, autoreactive T- and B-cell clones may be detected in the blood of normal individuals. There is no direct evidence, however, that cells directly involved in the pathogenesis of autoimmune diseases originate from these autoreactive clones. The presence of circulating autoreactive lymphocytes in healthy subjects must be considered as physiological. Indeed, tolerance during ontogenesis should not involve the removal of too many self-reactive clones. Due to the frequent molecular similarity between proteins of self and nonself, extensive deletion of potentially autoreactive lymphocytes recognizing autologous antigens would in fact cause a crippling reduction of the T- and B-cell repertoire.

Tolerance is ensured by several other peripheral mechanisms, which during a lifetime avoid the activation of self-reactive lymphocytes. An inherited impairment of suppressor mechanisms has been postulated, which allows escape of newly generated autoreactive clones. Although this issue has long been debated within the immunology community, several pieces of experimental evidence are now available which document the existence of T cells with immunomodulatory activity.

Molecular mimicry:

The number of amino acids from which proteins are made is relatively small and, even though the possible combinations are hundreds of thousands, identical stretches of sequence (less than 10 amino acids) are found relatively frequently among proteins of the body, as well as between self and nonself proteins. Moreover, several proteins are highly conserved phylogenetically, even among very distant species, probably because of their indispensable function within the organism. An immune response may be mounted against a microbial antigen that is similar or identical to a self antigen. The result will be an immune attack against the microorganism and the self tissue. A clinical example of disease caused by molecular mimicry is acute rheumatic fever, in which the antibody response mounted against a group A Streptococcus may cross-react with self antigens expressed on articular, cutaneous, cardiac and brain tissues, leading to the appearance of corresponding clinical manifestations (i.e. polyarthritis, erythema marginatum and subcutaneous nodules, carditis and chorea).

Abnormal presentation of self antigens:

Aberrant expression of major histocompatibility complex (MHC) class-II molecules:

In conditions of inflammation, the in situ release of cytokines (e.g. interferon gamma (IFNg)) may induce the expression of MHC class-II molecules on cells that do not usually express such molecules. This phenomenon may allow the presentation of yet unknown self antigens to autoreactive CD4+T cells. This theory is sustained by the evidence thatMHCclass-II molecules were expressed on B cells and capillaries around the islets of a pancreas from a child who died 24 h after the diagnosis of insulin-dependent diabetes. It was also shown that, upon viral infection or IFNg treatment, thyroid epithelial cells expressed MHC class-II molecules. This theory, although fascinating, lacks some corollaries that should explain why naiveTcells might migrate within a tissue where they are not expected to migrate, and how they become activated in the absence of costimulatory signals. Nevertheless, the aberrant expression of MHC class-II molecules within the tissue target of an autoimmune reaction might be responsible for an extension or aggravation of an autoimmune inflammatory process. Moreover, this model shifts the concept of autoimmunity from an abnormal T-cell response to an abnormal presentation of self antigens.

Binding of exogenous antigens to self antigens:

An autoantigen may become coupled to an exogenous antigen which acts as a carrier. In this case, CD4+ T cells specific for the exogenous antigen are activated and provide help to B cells specific for the self antigen. Activated B cells act as professional antigen-presenting cells and, by activating anticarrier T helper cells, perpetuate the autoreactive phenomenon. Moreover, owing to the complexity of the antigenic protein, a single carrier-specific CD4+ T-cell clone may help multiple B cells, each one specific for different epitopes within the autoantigen. This theory does not require a break of tolerance at the T-cell level, although it does require persistence of the source of carrier in the organism.

Overproduction of autoantigens:

Clonal deletion during ontogenesis is more likely to affect autoreactive clones with a high specificity for the antigen. Clones with low affinity for self epitopes may escape clonal deletion and reach the periphery, where they do not become activated because the autoantigens are not sufficiently concentrated to reach the threshold for cell activation. This immunological ignorance may be broken by the release of an excess of autoantigens in the presence of a milieu (e.g. inflammation), which ensures efficient processing and presentation of those autoantigens.

Disclosure of cryptic T-cell epitopes :

A protein is formed by several amino acid sequences which may represent T-cell epitopes. However, because of the complex mechanisms regulating the processing and presentation of T-cell epitopes, several sequences may act as immunodominant, whereas some others may be cryptic. The former will be readily recognized by T cells, whereas the latter will not, because even if presented they do not reach the threshold for T-cell activation. When this model is applied to thymic selection, it is obvious that the autoreactive T cells deleted during ontogenesis will be those specific for immunodominant epitopes. Autoreactive T-cell clones specific for cryptic epitopes and released from the thymus will be able to circulate freely and harmlessly unless a triggering event subverts the hierarchy of epitopes, and allows presentation of cryptic epitopes. This model received its first experimental support in the work by Gammon and Sercarz (1989). They demonstrated that T cells from adult mice rendered tolerant to whole lysozyme did not proliferate in response to immunization with the whole protein or peptides containing dominant determinants. Conversely, immunization with cryptic epitopes elicited a lysozyme-specific T-cell response.

Release of sequestered self antigens :

It is well known that immunologically privileged sites exist within the body (i.e. the brain, eye, testis and uterus), which are usually not patrolled by the sentinels of the immune system. However, once the barrier that hides these tissues is broken, they immediately become targets for autoimmune reactions. A classical example is sympathetic ophthalmia, which is an autoimmune inflammatory aggression to the contralateral eye of a subject who received an eye insult.

Epitope spreading:

The phenomenon of epitope spreading was first described by Lehmann et al., 1992, in a model of experimental allergic encephalomyelitis (EAE), which resembles the human disease multiple sclerosis. They showed that mice immunized with a single peptide epitope from the mouse myelin basic protein (MBP) in adjuvant developed a T-cell-proliferative response against the MBP protein, and EAE. A few weeks after immunization, T-cell-proliferative responses against other cryptic epitopes within theMBP were identified in the spleens of animalsimmunized with the single peptide.These findings suggested that, upon injection of a single T-cell epitope peptide, an MBP-specific CD4+ T-cell immune response was initiated, with release of MBP by damaged neuronal cells, and further processing and presentation of epitopes otherwise ignored. Therefore, irrespective of the nature of the mechanism that allows the presentation of a self epitope, once the self-specific immune response has been initiated it may spread to other self epitopes, previously ignored, for which the deletion of autoreactive T-cell clones is less likely to have occurred in the thymus.

Polyclonal lymphocyte activation:

T and B cells may be massively activated in the absence of a nominal antigen. An example is provided by bacterial lipopolysaccharides, which function as polyclonal B-cell activators. Another example is the infection by Epstein–Barr virus. Several autoimmune diseases (e.g. SLE and rheumatoid arthritis) are characterized by a polyclonal B-cell activation, confirmed by the presence of serum hypergammaglobulinaemia and positivity for rheumatoid factors (e.g. IgM reacting with the fragment crystallization (Fc) of IgG). Antigen-independent B-cell activation may also result from an inherited abnormality of B cells. Although polyclonal B-cell activation may be a relevant pathogenic mechanism in systemic autoimmune diseases, it does not seem to be involved in the pathogenesis of organspecific autoimmune diseases. See also: Epstein-Barr virus; Rheumatoid arthritis Polyclonal T-cell activation has also been hypothesized in the pathogenesis of autoimmune diseases. Several stimuli (superantigens, adjuvants) may activate a large number of T lymphocytes, among which autoreactive clones are nested. [25]

In general for mucocutaneous lesions include many of investigatory procedures. The commonest investigations include Nikolsky's sign. Pemphigus is classically associated with this sign other blistering conditions also exhibit this sign. Biopsy is another procedure done for almost all of the lesions. Punch biopsy is generally considered for the mucocutaneous lesions. Tzanck test is also a common test where sample is taken from a fresh vesicle and stained and tzanck cell is viewed. It is typical for mucocutaneous lesions. The current standard method for blistering mucocutaneous lesions is immunofluorescence. Both direct and indirect immunofluorescence are done. Radioimmunoassay was done before but due to the threat of radiation exposure to the patient ELISA is being done using enzymes as a immune sorbent assay. Its sensistivity and specificity is higher than all other procedures. In addition salt split technique is done. Culture is done to view microorganisms and LE inclusion test done specifically for lupus erythematosis. All these procedures provide us accurate diagnosis and helps the clinicians to treat the lesion appropriately.

A. INFECTIONS:

1) VIRAL:

i) HERPES SIMPLEX VIRUS:

ii) VARICELLA ZOSTER VIRUS:

iii) HAND-FOOT-AND-MOUTH DISEASE:

iv) HERPANGINA:

Viral culture has been the gold standard until recently, when PCR has become the diagnostic test for rapid and accurate enterovirus infection. The coxsackievirus can be cultured from stool and occasionally from skin vesicles. The virus grows well on human epithelial cell and monkey kidney cell culture. Laboratory confirmation can be made by virus isolation or by detection of serum antibodies. [11]

Typical clinical features will usually suffice to make a clinical diagnosis. However for definitive diagnosis cytological smears, antibody titers and viral isolation can be used.

Cytological smear requires deroofing a fresh vesicle, followed by scraping of the base of the lesion and the smear made should be stained with Papanicolaou's, Wright's or Giemsa's stain. The characteristic findings include the presence of multinucleated giant cells and intranuclear viral inclusion bodies such as Lipschütz bodies or Cowdry Type A (ovoid, amorphous, eosinophilic bodies that exhibit peri inclusion halo that is caused by the peripheral displacement of the nucleolus and the nuclear chromatin). The cells exhibit ballooning degeneration of the nucleus.

On biopsy the microscopic features include an ulcerated epithelium with large keratinocytes showing glassy giant marginated nuclei (Tzanck cells).

Alternatively viral isolation can be done. It is one of the most definitive methods of identifying HSV.

Serological tests can be used to detect antibodies in patient suffering from primary HSV. For the test, blood sample should be taken in the initial 3 days of an acute infection. Alternatively a convalescent blood sample can be obtained 4 weeks after the primary infection. It is believed that the antibody titer should increase by four times in convalescent serum sample for the diagnosis of the primary infection. [7]

14. BACTERIAL:

i) GONORRHOEA:

Rapid diagnosis is done by Gram staining of urethral discharge. Samples can be collected with Dacron or Rayon swabs. Special media used for gonococcus are Thayer-Martin media or Stuart or Armies media. [7]

The evidence of gram-negative diplococci in a Gram stained smear of exudates from the gonococcal lesions is suggestive of N. gonorrheae infection. [1]

ii) CAT SCRATCH DISEASE:

Neville and coworkers enumerated certain criteria for the diagnosis of cat-scratch fever. Evidence of at least three of the following four criteria is considered to be positive for cat-scratch disease:

1. Contact with a cat, presence of a scratch or a primary dermal or ocular lesion.
2. Positive Hangar–Rose skin test (cat-scratch disease skin test).

This skin test was first developed by Hanger and Rose in 1946. Aspirated material from a lymph node of a patient with known cat-scratch disease is pasteurized, standardized, and tested for sterility. It is then injected subdermally and skin reaction is noted.

3. Unidentifiable cause for lymphadenopathy.

4. Presence of pleomorphic bacilli with Warthin–Starry method or Brown–Hopps method.

However, serological test (ELISA for IgM antibodies to B. henselae) is the gold standard for the diagnosis of cat-scratch disease. Elevated serum titers are seen 1–3 weeks after the onset of the disease process. [7]

4) FUNGAL:

Histologic findings:

On histological section blastomyces can be easily discernible with PAS stain, H and E stain, PAP and methenamine silver stains. It can be cultured using Sabouraud's agar. [7]

5) CHLAMYDEAL:

Microscopic examination of Giemsa-stained films of pus or sections from a lymph node biopsy may demonstrate minute intracellular cocci. PCR, direct immunofluorescence, and culture of aspirated pus or lymph node biopsy material could be performed in specialized laboratories as serologic tests are less reliable. [8]

B. SKIN DISEASES:

1. PEMPHIGUS VULGARIS:

Tzanck's test:

The examination of fluid from a bulla (a blister) in search of Tzanck cells characteristic of varicella (chicken pox), herpes zoster, herpes simplex, and pemphigus vulgaris. It was named after a Russian dermatologist Arnault Tzanck (1886–1954). It is basically a type of exfoliative cytology. In pemphigus, acantholytic cells are seen and in herpes multinucleated giant cells with Lipschutz bodies are seen. [7]

CLINICAL EXAMINATION:

In patients with PV and active blistering, firm sliding pressure with a finger separates normal-looking epithelium (nikolsky's sign), but this is neither completely sensitive nor specific. [12]

BIOPSY:

Best done on intact vesicle or bulla less than 24hr old. Specimens taken from the advancing edge of the lesion where areas of characteristics SUPRABASILAR ACANTHOLYSIS is seen.

In P. VULGARIS, intercellular edema develops in epithelial cells, dissolution of intercellular bridges occurs, and the widening of intercellular spaces occurs which causes separation between cells and formation if blister above basal cell layer (supra basilar split). The present case showed typical histological features of intraepithelial blistering disorder with supraepithelial split and acantholytic cells. [12]

TZANK SMEAR:

The base of blister is scrapped and examined for acantholytic cells. The free floating rounded or ovoid acantholytic cells has an enlarged, hyperchromatic centrally or eccentrically situated nucleus. Basal cells are tightly attached to basal lamina but lose their attachment to one another, producing a TOMBSTONE appearance. Relatively fewer inflammatory cells are seen in P. vulgaris compared with other bullous diseases.[12]

COMPRESSED AIR TEST:

Application of a stream of compressed air to the oral mucous membrane
e of gingival tissues may cause a shimmering of the outer tissues followed by formation of bleb or a blister.[12]

IMMUNOFLORESENCE STUDIES:

The clinical diagnosis was always confirmed by direct and indirect immunofluorescence.

DIRECT IMMUNOFLORESENCE:

Fluorescence labeled antihuman immunoglobulins are placed over the patients tissue specimen. Circulating antibodies of IgG type, bound to the intercellular cement region of the oral mucosa were detected. In case of PV the technique will detect antibodies usually IgG & compliment bound to the surface of Keratinocytes.

INDIRECT IMMUNOFLORESENCE:

Serum from a patient is placed over a prepared slide of an epidermal structure (usually monkey oesophagus). The slide is then overlaid with flouroscein tagged antihuman gama globulin. Patient with PV have antikeratinocyte antibodies against intercellular substance that show up under a fluorescent microscope. The titer of antibody has been directly related to level of clinical disease. The test distinguishes pemphigus from pemphigoid & other chronic oral lesions. [12]

UPPER GASTROINTESTINAL ENDOSCOPY:

May be useful in identifying oesophageal involvement. [12]

ELISA:

Can detect Dsg1 & Dsg3 (Desmoglein) in serum samples. [12]

IMMUNOPRECIPITATION AND IMMUNOELECTRON MICROSCOPY:

The targeted antigen recognised by autoantibodies is 130KD glycoprotein identical to Desmoglein. [12]

2) BULLOUS PEMPHIGOID:

IMMUNOFLUORESCENT TECHNIQUES:

Direct Immunofluorescence (DIF):

DIF is a one-step procedure that involves application of fluoresceinated antibodies to a frozen section of the skin. [25] DIF is diagnostic in pemphigus, pemphigoid, gestational pemphigoid, dermatitis herpatiformis, linear IgA bullous dermatosis, and epidermolysis bullosa acquisita.

Indirect Immunofluorescence (IDIF):

IDIF is a two-step procedure in which patient smear is layered on the substrate followed by the application of fluoresceinated antibodies. IDIF of the patient's serum can be used as a screening test for circulating antibodies mainly IgG and IgA. IDIF on monkey or guinea pig esophagus has become an established mode of testing for serum antibody in pemphigus; whereas for the subepidermal autoimmune blistering diseases, the preferred substrate is normal human skin that has been split with 1 M sodium chloride solution. [3]

SALT SPLIT TECHNIQUE:

The purpose of this procedure is to differentiate between two immunobullous skin disease having similar features clinically, on histology and on routine DIF, that is, bullous pemphigoid and epidermolysis bullosa acquisita. Apart from these two lesions, also list the findings of salt split technique in other VB lesions. Punch biopsy samples were incubated in 5 ml of NaCl (1 mol/L) at 4°C for 24 h. The epidermis was then teased from the dermis with the use of a fine forceps. The specimens were then processed in the same manner and treated with IgG and C3 conjugates as in DIF. Salt split technique is of two types: Direct and indirect. Direct technique is performed on patient skin biopsy that is either freshly taken or on the one that has previously been investigated by routine DIF; whereas in indirect technique, a sample of normal human skin is used as a substrate, after artificially inducing the junctional split, cryocut sections are prepared, and then IDIF with patient's serum is carried out. Prior to DIF, salt splitting of the patient's skin results in linear deposition of basement membrane zone immunoreactants to the roof, floor, or both. The binding of immunoreactants to hemidesmosomal and upper lamina lucida antigens results in roof or epidermal pattern; whereas, binding of immunoreactants to lower lamina lucida and sublamina densa results in a floor or dermal pattern. Prior to IDIF techniques, cleavage of normal skin is performed with 1mM phenylmethylsulfonyl fluoride (PMSF). This enzyme inhibitor ensures complete preservation of antigenic structures in the substrate, thus helps in the differentiation of subepidermal blistering diseases whether the sera binds either to the roof or floor of the split substrate. [3]

3) MUCOUS MEMBRANE PEMPHIGOID:

Microscopic Appearance:

The intact epithelium detaches cleanly from the underlying connective tissue. There is often chronic inflammation in the connective tissue, but this is sometimes subtle or absent.

Immunofluorescence Pattern:

Direct immunofluorescence shows a linear deposit of IgG, IgA, C3 or a combination of these in the BMZ. Circulating autoantibodies are usually low in concentration although often sufficient to show linear BMZ staining by indirect immunofluorescence on either the epithelial or connective tissue surface. [14]

4) LUPUS ERYTHEMATOSUS:

LE cell inclusion phenomenon or LE test:

This test was first explained by Hargraves for systemic LE (SLE). In tissues, nuclei of damaged cells react with antinuclear antibodies (ANAs), lose their chromatin pattern and become homogenous to produce LE or hematoxylin bodies (amorphous round body in the cytoplasm of the cell). If the serum from a patient suffering from SLE is added to the buffy coat of normal blood, a typical LE cell will develop. LE cell is any phagocytic leukocyte (neutrophils or macrophage) that has engulfed the denatured nucleus of an injured cell and contains an amorphous round body (LE body), serum nuclear globulin (IgG), and complement. [3]

5) DERMATITIS HERPETIFORMIS:

Dermatitis herpetiformis is the cutaneous manifestation of celiac disease (sprue). In celiac disease, there are typically autoantibodies against endomysium and tissue transglutaminase; additional autoantibodies against epidermal transglutaminase are responsible for the cutaneous signs of the disease. [26]

6. ORAL LICHEN PLANUS:

The diagnosis of LP is based on the clinical presentationand should be confirmed by biopsy, if suspected. Histopathology is often conclusive, but in vesiculobullous CLP or erosive OLP, direct immunofluorescence (DIF) studies can be an integral step in differentiating between LP and other diseases. DIF typically demonstrates globular IgM deposition at the dermal-epidermal junction in LP. Although the existence of fibrin deposition at the mucosal submucosal interface and within vessels and the presence of colloid bodies is highly sensitive for a diagnosis of LP, it lacks specificity. Indirect immunofluorescence and enzymelinked immunosorbent assays can also be helpful in reaching a diagnosis. [12]

7) ERYTHEMA MULTIFORME:

A diagnosis of EM can be difficult to readily establish, and there can be a need to differentiate from viral stomatitides, pemphigus, TEN and the subepithelial immune blistering disorders (pemphigoid and others). There are no specific diagnostic tests for EM and the diagnosis is mainly clinical supported if necessary by biopsy. Biopsy of perilesional tissue, with histological and immunostaining examination are essential if a specific diagnosis is required. Biopsy shows intraepithelial edema and spongiosis early on, with satellite cell necrosis (individual eosinophilic necrotic keratinocytes surrounded by lymphocytes), vacuolar degeneration of the junctional zone and severe papillary edema with sub- or intra-epithelial vesiculation, and intense lymphocytic infiltration and immune deposits of fibrin and C3 at the basement membrane zone. There may be a perivascular lymphocytic infiltrate (CD4+ more than CD8+ T lymphocytes) with a few neutrophils and occasional eosinophils, and perivascular IgM, C3 and fibrin deposits. However, pathology can be variable and immunostaining is not specific for EM.

In EM major a complete blood count, urea and electrolytes, erythrocyte sedimentation rate (ESR), liver function tests, and cultures from blood, sputum and erosive areas should be taken. To identify an etiological agent it may be helpful to undertake serology for HSV or M. pneumoniae, or other micro-organisms. [6]

8) TOXIC EPIDERMAL NECROLYSIS (TEN):

Diagnosis of toxic epidermal necrolysis Sheet-like loss of the epithelium and a positive Nikolsky sign are characteristic. Biopsy of perilesional tissue, with histological and immunostaining examination are essential to the diagnosis. Histopathologic examination is characteristic showing necrosis of the whole epithelium detached from the lamina propria. [6]

9) EPIDERMOLYSIS BULLOSA:

Patients with epidermolysis bullosa acquisita develop antibodies against type VII collagen (6), with the NC1 domain as the immune-dominant region (e41). [26]

10) DYSKERATOSIS CONGENITA:

Histologic Findings:

Skin biopsy specimens from the areas of reticulated pigmentation typically show mild hyperkeratosis, epidermal atrophy, telangiectasia of the superficial blood vessels, and melanophages in the papillary dermis. Interface changes have also been reported, with mild basal layer vacuolization and a lymphocytic inflammatory infiltrate in the upper dermis. Oral lesions have not been thoroughly studied but the leukoplakic lesions appear to be nonspecific hyperparakeratosis or hyperorthokeratosis and acanthosis. Depending on the stage of the disease, the epithelium may show dysplasia. The exact nature of the preceding vesicles and ulcers has not been described.

Laboratory Findings:

Many cases have been characterized also by hematologic changes including anemia, leukopenia, thrombocytopenia and pancytopenia. Some patients have developed Fanconi's anemia. In fact, the suggestion has been made that Fanconi's syndrome, or Fanconi's familial pancytopenia, is simply a varied expression of dyskeratosis congenita. [1]

C) DRUG INDUCED:

1) LICHENOID REACTION:

Diagnosis:

There is no specific test for the diagnosis of LR. The widely accepted criterion is based on the observation of disappearance of the lesions after withdrawal of triggering agent and recurrence of the lesions when they are reintroduced. [1]

2) PEMPHIGUS FOLIACEUS:

Nikolsky's test:

It was first described by Piotr Vasiliyevich Nikolsky (1858-1940) a Russian dermatologist. He related how, after rubbing the skin of patients who had pemphigus foliaceous, there was a blistering or denudation of the epidermis with a glistening, moist surface underneath. According to his explanation, the skin showed a weak relationship and contact between the corneal and granular cell layers on all surfaces and even in places between lesions (e.g. blisters, excoriations) on seemingly unaffected skin. Nikolsky's observations were later confirmed by Lyell in 1956, who described a Nikolsky's sign in patients with toxic epidermal necrolysis.

It is characteristically seen in intraepidermal bullous disorders; whereas in subepidermal VB diseases, the sign is generally absent. Nikolsky's sign is classically associated with pemphigus vulgaris. However, other blistering conditions are also known to exhibit this sign including pemphigus foliaceous, paraneoplastic pemphigus, oral lichen planus, mucous membrane pemphigoid, bullous pemphigoid, epidermolysis bullosa, Stevens-Johnson Syndrome, Staphylococcal scalded skin syndrome (SSSS), toxic epidermal necrolysis (TEN), linear IgA disease, lupus erythematous (LE), dermatomyositis, chronic erythema multiforme and graft-versus-host disease.

This test is difficult to produce in the oral cavity as the blisters and vesicles rupture very early. A Nikolsky sign in the oral cavity is said to be positive when tissue ulceration or blistering is seen after applying mucosal pressure either by blowing air or using a blunt instrument or finger.

Principle:

In patients with active blistering, firm sliding pressure with a finger separates normal appearing epidermis, producing erosion.

Method:

This is done by applying lateral pressure with the index finger which provides the shearing force to disrupt the intercellular adhesion in clinical Nikolsky's sign. If the weakening of the intercellular adhesion is present but not marked, then the same shearing force may produce minimal damage at the cellular level which can be demonstrated only microscopically. As microscopic Nikolsky's sign sometimes spans only a few cells, serial sections may be required to avoid missing a cleavage. [3]

3) DRUG INDUCED ERYTHEMA MULTIFORME:

The mechanisms of tissue damage in EM appear to differ between virally-induced and drug-induced EM. In drug induced erythema multiforme, the reactive metabolites of the initiating drug induce the disease. T cells do not produce IFN-γ in drug induced lesions but rather the lesions are characterized by TNF-α present in keratinocytes, macrophages and monocytes. In contrast, TNF- α has not been detected in EM and it has even been proposed that its presence may be used as a laboratory test to distinguish drug-induced lesions from EM. In EM tissue damage appears to be the result of delayed type hypersensitivity. [9]

4) DRUG INDUCED LINEAR Ig A DISEASE:

Laboratory Findings:

Routine histology demonstrates a subepithelial lesion in the basement membrane similar to MMP, but DIF study will show deposition of I gA rather than I gG. II F is usually negative, but when positive, it will demonstrate circulating IgA antibodies against a basement membrane antigen. [8]

5) DRUG-INDUCED MELANOSIS:

If the onset of the melanosis can be temporally and accurately associated with use of a specific medication (frequently within several weeks or months before development of the pigmentation), then no further intervention is warranted. In most cases, the discoloration tends to fade within a few months after the drug is discontinued. Pigmentation associated with hormone therapy may tend to persist for longer periods of time, despite discontinuation of the medications.

A differential diagnosis includes other causes of diffuse mucosal pigmentation. Laboratory tests may be necessary to rule out an underlying endocrinopathy. [8]

If the mucocutaneous lesion involves the presence of microbes antiviral drugs (like acyclovir), antibacterial (like gentamicin) and antifungal (like itraconazole) are prescribed accordingly. The formost therapy suggested for oral mucocutaneous lesion is complete periodontal makeover and maintenance of good oral hygiene. Maintenance of oral hygiene involves proper brushing and usage of 0.2% of aqueous solution of chlorhexidine mouth wash. For mucocutaneous lesions at first topical corticosteroids are preferred. In addition corticosteroids are preferred such as prednisolone etc. These corticosteroids are used in combination with systemic corticosteroids in severe cases. Immunosuppressive agents like cyclosporine and azathrioprine are also used in combination with the corticosteroids for autoimmune diseases. Oral antacids are also prescribed in cases of ulcers. Newer drugs are also prescribed like rituximab.

A. INFECTIONS:

1) VIRAL:

i) HERPES SIMPLEX VIRUS:

Treatment of primary herpetic gingivostomatitis may include the use of systemic anti-viral therapy as well as palliative measures for relief of discomfort. Oral acyclovir is useful in reducing viral shedding; however, it does not always alter the clinical course of the disease. As a result, palliative therapy may be necessary. Topically-applied oral rinses containing an anesthetic solution may provide temporary pain relief. Analgesics and antipyretics are often indicated, and care must be taken to insure adequate fluid intake to prevent dehydration. Treatment of recurrent herpetic lesions may include the use of systemic and/or topically-applied acyclovir.104-106 Orally-administered lysine has been reported to interfere with viral replication and has shown limited therapeutic benefit in some clinical trials. [10]

ii) VARICELLA ZOSTER VIRUS:

Vaccination against varicella zoster should be given to infants between 12th and 18th months of life. The management of the disease is mainly symptomatic. Acyclovir can be administered in the early phases of the disease. [7]

iii) HAND-FOOT-AND-MOUTH DISEASE:

Topical application of anesthetics like viscous lidocaine and diphenhydramine may be used to manage painful oral ulcers. Sucralfate suspension can also be effectively used. Fever and arthralgias can be treated using antipyretics and analgesics. Literature review reveals that there is a reported quickerresolution of symptoms with the use of oral acyclovir. A low intensity laser ablation of the oral ulcers is said to shorten the duration of painful oral ulcers. [7]

iv) HERPANGINA:

Herpangina is a self-limiting disease. The fever associated with this condition usually subsides within 3–4 days. The oral ulcers heal within a week. The condition can be managed symptomatically with antipyretics and analgesic/ anesthetic mouthrinses. [7]

2) BACTERIAL:

i) IMPETIGO:

Impetigo is a self-limiting condition and it usually resolves spontaneously in about 2 weeks without scar formation. The topical antibiotics mupirocin and fusidic acid are effective. Orally administered systemic antibiotics can be used in severe forms of the condition. [7]

ii) GONORRHOEA:

Oropharyngeal gonorrhea is best managed with intramuscular injection of ceftriaxone. Other drugs that have been used effectively include cefixime and ciprofloxacin. [7]

iii) CAT SCRATCH DISEASE:

The condition is self-limiting and usually resolves in about 6 months duration. Suppurative nodes may be aspirated to evacuate the pus. The recommended surgical procedure to evacuate the pus is to introduce the needle into the skin 1 to 2 cm away from the swelling

and then burrow beneath the surface of the skin to reach the affected node. The technique helps to hasten the healing and prevent formation of a persistent sinus.
Antibiotics such as gentamicin, penicillin, ciprofl oxacin and rifampin may be used when systemic involvement is apparent. [7]

3) FUNGAL:

For mild cases itraconazole and ketoconazole can be used effectively. Patients who are refractory to ketoconazole can be treated with amphotericin B. [7]

4) CHLAMYDEAL:

Tetracycline, chloramphenicol, streptomycin garamycin, and cotrimoxazole are effective in the treatment of this disease. Complete healing usually occurs within two to three weeks. It has been noted that, after treatment, improvement of the genital lesions is usually accompanied by improvement of the extragenital oral lesion; conversely, exac-erbation of genital lesions usually results in worsening of the oral condition. [1]

B) SKIN DISEASES:

1. PEMPHIGUS VULGARIS:

TREATMENT MEASURES:

Periodontal therapy is an essential part of overall treatment of pemphigus. Optimal oral hygiene is important because the gingival involvement may present an exaggereted response to bacterial plaque.

Oral lesions are difficult to treat because of trauma to the surface epithelium whenever the patient eats.

DIET CONSIDERATIONS -

Patients on steroid therapy are monitored for weight gain and advised low salt, low fat, low calorie diet. Also advised increased consumption of potassium and protein rich meals. Corticosteroids form the mainstay of treatment in Pemphigus cases. In patients with P. vulgaris there is pronounced imbalance of helper T – T suppressor ratio, which is restored by corticosteroid therapy. Oral lesions of Pemphigus Vulgaris may respond partially to topical or intralesional corticosteroids. Systemic corticosteroids. (1-2 mg/kg/day) remain the mainstay of therapy of patients with oral lesions. Corticosteroids with less adverse effects are preferred.

In cases of severe disease 80mg daily Prednosolone may be used. Combining corticosteroids (Prednisolone or prednisone) with immune-suppressive agents, such as cyclosporine, methotexate, azathioprine and cyclophosphamide makes it possible to use much smaller doses of the corticosteroids and thereby reduces the chance for steroid- related complications. Dapsone has been used in treating cutaneous pemphigus vulgaris. Plasminogen activator may have a role in pemphigus, drugs such as Tranexamic acid, which prevents con version of Plasminogen to Plasmin may be effective in treating

Pemphigus.

Plasmapheresis: is done with cyclosporin or cyclophosphamide. This process removes circulating antibodies. It affects B cell proliferation. Plasmapheresis has been used in patients who are refractory to therapy with steroids in doses of 2mg/kg/day. The low levels of antibodies resulting from plasmapheresis cause a rebound effect where new antibodies are produced in excess of the original levels. However, this rebound effect can be controlled by administration of an immunosuppressive agent.

Photopheresis: where in WBC's are photoinactivated with methoxsalen and UV-A in an extra corporeal system.

PUVA: Administration of 8-MethoxyPsoralen followed by exposure of peripheral blood to Ultraviolet radiation. Intravenous Pulse therapy of corticosteroids- IV methyl Prednisolone 1gm daily/5days. Intravenous Immunoglobulins: Proved successful & safe in steroid resistant PV57

Newer drugs:

- Cholinergic agonists (modulates autoimmune response which require autoreactive helper T cells that regulate IgG isotope switching)
- Rituximab (Anti CD20 monoclonal antibody)
- Proteinase inhibitors
- Chimergic molecules (for specific recognition & elimination of autoimmune B cells targeting Dsg3 specific T cells). [12]

2) BULLOUS PEMPHIGOID:

Bullous pemphigoid is treated with systemic steroids. Azathioprine and cyclophosphamide have also been used successfully. [7]

3) MUCOUS MEMBRANE PEMPHIGOID:

Patients with involvement of the conjunctiva and pharyngeal, laryngeal and genital mucosa should be referred to appropriate medical personnel for therapy, which is usually more aggressive than that for patients with oral lesions only.

Patients who exhibit only mild oral lesions may require no treatment, as the risk of therapeutic side effects outweighs the benefit of the treatment. Many patients develop a tolerance to the oral lesions and cease complaining about oral discomfort despite the persistence of mild disease.

Because the disease is considered autoimmune, the first line of treatment for those with only oral lesions is the use of topical corticosteroids, such as fluocinonide. However, this treatment often fails. Periodic bursts of systemic corticosteroids, such as prednisone, may achieve success in some patients, whereas others notice no improvement.14 Patients resistant to corticosteroid therapy may benefit from dapsone (avlosulfone) therapy or combined tetracycline and nicotinamide therapy.

Recently, topical tacrolimus has been used experimentally with some success on a patient with genital lesions.

Cyclophosphamide, azathioprine and methotrexate are used in combination with systemic corticosteroids in severe cases. Intravenous immunoglobulin (IVIG) has been tried with some success. In some patients, any combination of treatments is unsuccessful, and these patients may continue to suffer unabated for decades. In all cases involving the gingiva, excellent oral hygiene to reduce bacterial plaque is recommended, despite the pain and potential blistering associated with brushing. [14]

4) LUPUS ERYTHEMATOSUS:

The basis of treatment is the use of corticosteroids, given in a dose adequate to control the multisystem disease and to return the anti-DNA antibodies and complement levels to normal.

Depending on the severity and nature of the disease the dose of corticosteroids can vary from 10 mg to 1 g intravenously per day.

In patients with repeated exacerbations of the disease at moderately high doses of corticosteroids, azathioprine may be useful to allow the patient to be maintained on lower doses of corticosteroids. Antimalarial drugs are useful in patients with skin abnormalities, alopecia or mucosal ulcers. In the recent times, severe and unresponsive cases have been managed successfully with plasmapheresis or leukapheresis.

Dental considerations:

1. Platelet count estimation may be required prior to any oral surgical procedure, to evaluate the severity of thrombocytopenia.
2. Bacterial endocarditis—Libman–Sacks vegetations may be found under mitral valve leaflets in SLE. These vegetations rarely affect function but can lead to bacterial endocarditis. Patients with SLE have to be considered for antibiotic prophylaxis before dental treatment that is likely to cause bacteremia.
3. According to Roura et al (1991), drugs that have a photosensitizing potential like penicillin, sulphonamides and NSAIDs should be used judiciously as they tend to exacerbate SLE.
4. SLE patients are susceptible to shock and infection as they are medicated with adrenal suppressing doses of corticosteroids or cytotoxic drugs. [7]

5) DERMATITIS HERPETIFORMIS:

Management:

Dermatitis herpetiformis usually runs a prolonged course and sometimes persists for life. Patients are advised to avoid gluten in the diet. Dapsone is usually the drug of choice. In the initial stages 50 mg/day is given and later increased to about 300 mg/day as per the requirement. [7]

6. ORAL LICHEN PLANUS:

In general, nonerosive oral lichen planus is asymptomatic and treatment is often unnecessary. However, patients with erosive type oral lichen planus often present with significant management problems. At present, none of the available treatment is specific or universally effective.

An algorithm for the management of oral lichen planus is shown.

All patients should optimize their oral hygiene. Oral candidiasis should be excluded or treated accordingly. In symptomatic patients with apparent contact dental factor, patch test with replacement of the amalgam or gold restorative material is suggested in those who are sensitized to these metals. In those with no apparent contact factor, topical or intralesional steroid is usually the first line treatment. A short course of systemic steroid may be necessary for more rapid control. In steroid dependent patients, azathioprine or topical cyclosporine can be added as an adjunctive therapy. In refractory cases, alternative therapies such as topical or systemic retinoids, antimalarial, dapsone, oral PUVA, thalidomide or topical tacrolimus may be considered. Surgical treatments such as laser, cryotherapy and excision may exacerbate the conditions due to the Koebner phenomenon. [6]

7) ERYTHEMA MULTIFORME:

Spontaneous healing of EM can be slow upto 2–3 weeks in minor and upto 6 weeks in major EM. Treatment is thus, indicated but controversial (Katz, et al. 1999). No specific treatment is available but supportive care is important; a liquid diet and intravenous fluid therapy may be necessary. Early ophthalmological and dermatological consultation is needed for diagnosis and management. Precipitating factors, when identified, should be treated Antimicrobials may be indicated, acyclovir in EM or tetracycline in EM related to M. pneumoniae. A 5-day course of acyclovir at the first sign of lesions, or 400 mg qds for 6 months is useful for prophylaxis in EM. Continuous therapy of valacyclovir, 500 mg twice a day, has also been reported to be effective.

The use of corticosteroids is controversial. Minor EM may respond to topical corticosteroids, though systemic corticosteroids may be required and patients with major EM or SJS may need to be admitted for hospital care and should be treated with systemic corticosteroids (prednisolone 0.5–1.0 mg/kg)/day) tapered over 7–10 days) and/or azathioprine or other immunomodulatory drugs. 50% of SJS patients in one series required supplemental hydration or alimentation because of the severity of the oral cavity involvement

Other treatments used, may include cyclophosphamide, dapsone, cyclosporine, azathioprine, levamisole and thalidomide. Plasmapheresis possibly has a place in the management of severe disease. Oral antacids may be helpful for management of discrete oral ulcers. Electrolytes and nutritional support should be started as soon as possible. Oral hygiene should be improved with 0.2% aqueous chlorhexidine mouthwash. [6]

8) TOXIC EPIDERMAL NECROSIS:

The offending drug should be immediately identified and discontinued. The following treatment guidelines followed by University of Florida can be practiced effectively. University of Florida management guidelines for TEN and SJS

1. Admit patient directly to the burn intensive care unit (BICU) or an intensive care setting
2. Discontinue corticosteroids if they are being used to treat the eruption
3. Discontinue unnecessary medications and suspect medications
4. Obtain baseline laboratory tests, such as complete blood count, liver function tests, metabolic panel, chest radiographs, and any other appropriate imaging or serologic tests, including an immediate (stat) immunoglobulin A (IgA) serum level
5. Look carefully for evidence of infection
6. Obtain punch biopsies of skin for diagnosis confirmation. An alternative for rapid diagnosis is removal of a bulla roof for immediate frozen sections to differentiate between TEN and staphylococcal scalded skin syndrome (SSSS)
7. Culture skin, blood, body orifices (as appropriate), and urine daily to monitor for early infection, and keep abreast of changing antibiotic sensitivities
8. Use systemic antibiotics only for documented infections or signs of sepsis
9. Place large-bore intravenous lines or a central venous line in an area of uninvolved skin to ensure adequate intravenous access
10. If within 48–72 hours of bulla onset, use intravenous immunoglobulin (IVIG), sucrose depleted, 1 g/kg/day for 3 days infused over 4 hours. If 72 hours have passed, but the patient is still actively progressing with new lesions, IVIG may still be useful
11. Monitor fluid and electrolytes closely and begin total parenteral nutrition (TPN) in patients unable to take nourishment. Fluid replacement need not be as aggressive as for burns of same extent
12. Debridement of necrotic and desquamating areas may be performed
13. Consult ophthalmologist to assess ocular involvement
14. Consult otorhinolaryngologist to evaluate extent of upper respiratory tract involvement

15. Further consultations driven by patient condition (i.e. internal medicine to manage comorbidities, pulmonary medicine for airway involvement, gastroenterology for alimentary involvement, and gynecology or urology for genitourinary involvement)
16. Physical therapy daily to preserve limb mobility
17. Pain relief measures, such as patient-controlled analgesia (PCA) pump
18. Hydrotherapy (whirlpool) if needed
19. Non-stick dressings to denuded areas, saturated with 0.5% silver nitrate impregnated every 3–8 hour as needed. Pre-impregnated dressings with silver nitrate are an alternative.
20. Avoid sulfa-containing topical or systemic preparations
21. Oral care with chlorhexidine rinses and white petrolatum to lips
22. Air-fluidized bed to minimize shearing force
23. Keep room warm to prevent hypothermia
24. Foley catheter and nasogastric tube placement only when necessary
25. Avoid unnecessary manipulation of skin. Adhesive tape should not be applied directly to involved skin when possible
26. Baby shampoo for cleansing hairy areas daily
27. Mineral oil or petrolatum for dry skin
28. Skin substitute grafting (porcine xenografts or artificial skin) based on BICU protocol. [7]

9) EPIDERMOLYSIS BULLOSA:

This group of diseases cannot be cured so that therapy is chiefly symptomatic. The simplex form of the disease requires little treatment; the lethal form will terminate fatally in most cases regardless of management. In the dystrophic forms prevention of trauma may reduce the incidence of bulla formation, but this is almost impossible to achieve. Antibiotics are useful in controlling secondary infection and cortisteroids have sometimes been found effective. EB is a lifelong disease. Some subtypes, specially the milder EB forms, improve with age. [6]

10) DYSKERATOSIS CONGENITA:

Management:

Pancytopenia responds to androgen therapy in about 50% of patients. Supportive care is important. Bone marrow transplant has cured about 25% of a small number of patients. Oral leukoplakia should be treated conventionally.

Dental considerations:

It is imperative to test blood coagulation values before proceeding with surgery in patients with aplastic anemia and pancytopenia. [7]

C) DRUG INDUCED:

1) LICHENOID REACTION:

Treatment and Prognosis:

Identification and elimination of the triggering factors play a major role in the management of LR. Lichenoid lesions can take many months or longer to resolve. As per Haute and coworkers, the malignant transformation rate is reportedly higher in oral lichenoid lesions which do not have all the typical clinical and histologic features of oral lichen planus. [1]

2) PEMPHIGUS FOLIACEUS:

It is well known that drug-induced pemphigus can follow two different courses after withdrawal of drugs. If the disease continues despite drug withdrawal, it is called "drug-triggered pemphigus", whereas the form that resolves upon discontinuation of the culprit drug is called "drug-induced pemphigus". Permanent recovery from the disease after withdrawal of the culprit drug, also favored by short courses of steroid therapy, suggests that in these patients, the acantholysis is induced by drug with a "biochemical mechanism", and thus in the absence of autoantibodies. [27]

3) DRUG INDUCED ERYTHEMA MULTIFORME:

Identification of the cause should be made if possible. If a drug is suspected, it must be withdrawn. Infections should be appropriately treated after cultures and/or serologic tests have been performed. For all forms of EM, symptomatic treatment, including oral antihistamines, analgesics, local skin care, and soothing mouthwashes, is of great importance. Topical steroids may be considered. Oral antacids may be helpful for discrete oral ulcers. The use of liquid antiseptics, such as 0.05% chlorhexidine, during bathing is preferable.

Systemic corticosteroids are controversial, and some believe they may predispose to complications. [1]

4) DRUG INDUCED LINEAR IgA DISEASE:

The lesions of LABD generally follow a chronic course with periods of acute exacerbations. Spontaneous remission may be seen in some patients. However almost all patients exhibit recurrence. Dermal lesions are managed with dapsone or sulfapyridine. However mucosal lesions are usually refractory to dapsone. Prednisolone along with dapsone will usually help in controlling the condition. Lewis et al (2007) successfully treated a patient suffering from LABD with oral mucosal involvement using mycophenolate, an antiproliferative immunosuppressive agent. They reported that mycophenolate can be used as a useful adjunct to manageoral lesions of LABD, when other immunosuppressants are contraindicated. [7]

5) DRUG-INDUCED MELANOSIS:

Treatment and prognosis:

Although the discolorations of the oral mucosa may be aesthetically displeasing, they cause no long-term problems. In most instances, discontinuing the medication results in gradual fading of the areas of hyperpigmentation. [18]

BIBLIOGRAPHY:

1. Shafer, Hine, Levi. Shafer's textbook of oral pathology.7th edition. Elsevier publications.

2. Yasmeen J Bhat, Saima Aleem, Iffat Hassan, and Sheikh Manzoor. Oral Manifestations of Dermatological Disorders: Journal of Medical and Health Sciences 2014 July - September; 3 (3): 4-13.

3. Varun Rastogi, Rachna Sharma, Satya Ranjan Misra, Lalita Yadav. Diagnostic procedures for autoimmune vesiculobullous diseases: J Oral Maxillofac Pathol. 2014 Sep-Dec; 18(3): 390–397.

4. Subramaniyam. Classification of oral lesions 2009: 8. www.oralpath.org.in

5. Burcu SENGÜVEN et al. Oral mucosal lesions: a retrospective review of one institution's 13-year experience Turkish Journal of Medical Sciences. Turk J Med Sci 2015 Feb 9. 45: 241-245.

6. Vijay Kumar Biradar. Mucocutaneous Lesions in Dentistry: Jaypee Brothers Medical Publishers.

7. Ravikiran Ongole, Praveen B N. Textbook of Oral Medicine Oral Diagnosis and Oral Radiology. Elseiver Publications. 2nd edition

8. Greenberg, Glick, Ship. Burket's Oral medicine. 11th edition. Decker .2008

9. Sangeetha and Dhayanand John Victor. The molecular aspects of oral mucocutaneous diseases: International Journal of Genetics and Molecular Biology. 2011 November; 3(10). 141-148.

10. Oral Features of Mucocutaneous Disorders Committee on Research, Science and Therapy. The American Academy of Periodontology Scientific, Clinical and Educational Affairs Department. 1994 April.

11. Sridhar Reddy Erugula et al. Vesiculobullous lesions of the oral cavity. International Archives of Integrated Medicine, 2016 November; 3 (11) 154-163.

12. Shamimul Hasan. Oral signs in Mucocutaneous Disorders - Report of three cases and Review of Literature. Recent Researches in Medicine and Medical Chemistry.

13. Sridevi P, Munisekhar MS, Harika CH, Rama Krishna A. Oral Manifestations of Autoimmune Diseases. International Journal of Oral & Maxillofacial Pathology. 2012; 3(4):27-33.

14. Mark R. Darling, Tom Daley. Blistering Mucocutaneous Diseases of the Oral Mucosa — A Review:
Part 1. Mucous Membrane Pemphigoid. J Can Dent Assoc 2005; 71(11):851–854.

15. Farzam Gorouhi, Parastoo Davari, and Nasim Fazel. Cutaneous and Mucosal Lichen Planus: A Comprehensive Review of Clinical Subtypes, Risk Factors, Diagnosis, and Prognosis. Scientific World Journal Volume 2014, 1-22.

16. EVERSOLE-Contemporary Oral and Maxillofacial Pathology second edition 0-323-01723-1. Copyright 2004, Mosby, Inc. All rights reserved.

17. James W. Little, Donald A. Falace, Craig S. Miller, Nelson L. Rhodus.
Dental management Medically Compromised Patients: 8th edition. Elsevier publications. China. 2013.

18. Neville, Damm, Allen, Bouquot. Oral and Maxillofacial Pathology. Elsevier publications. 3rd edition.

19. Pablo Demelo-Rodríguez, Norberto Ortego-Centeno, Jose Luis Callejas-Rubio Groove sign. European Journal of Internal Medicine 2015. Elsevier publications. November 14; 3–4.

20. George Laskaris. Laskaris-Pocket Atlas of Oral Diseases. 2006 Thieme. 2nd edition.

21 Regezi, Scuibba, Jordan. Oral Pathology Clinical Pathologic Correlation. 6th edition. Elsevier Publication. 2012.

22. Foliaceus. Kirk A. James, Donna A. Culton, Luis A. Diaz. Diagnosis & Clinical Features of Pemphigus. Dermatol Clin. 2011 July; 29(3): 405–412.

23. Fransesca Angiero, Stefano Benedicenti, Rolando Crippa, Sarah Magistro, Davide Farronato and Michele Stefani. A Rare Case of Desquamative Gingivitis due to Linear IgA Disease: Morphological and Immunofluorescence Features. In vivo 2007 21; 1093-1098.

24. Nita Chainani. Oral manifestations of autoimmune blistering diseases - clinical presentation.

25. Matteo Bellone. Autoimmune Disease: Pathogenesis ENCYCLOPEDIA OF LIFE SCIENCES. 2005, John Wiley & Sons publications.

26. Enno Schmidt, Detlef Zillikens. The Diagnosis and Treatment of Autoimmune Blistering Skin Diseases: Dtsch Arztebl Int 2011; 108(23): 399–405.

Table of contents

FSC
www.fsc.org
MIX
Papier | Fördert
gute Waldnutzung
FSC® C083411

Kolibri 360 GmbH
Ferdinand-Jühlke-Straße 7
99095 Erfurt, Deutschland
produktsicherheit@kolibri360.de

Druck:
CPI Druckdienstleistungen GmbH
im Auftrag der
Kolibri 360 GmbH
Ferdinand-Jühlke-Str. 7
99095 Erfurt